Praise for *Reclaiming Body Trust*

"*Reclaiming Body Trust* is a compassionate, inclusive book that provides vital vocabulary and a framework for those seeking to understand and heal their relationship with their body. Using real-life narratives and their own extensive clinical experience, the authors have created a superb resource that will be life-changing for all who read it."

—Jennifer L. Gaudiani, MD, CEDS-S, FAED, founder and director of the Gaudiani Clinic and author of *Sick Enough: A Guide to the Medical Complications of Eating Disorders*

"Healing from the trauma of diet culture, body commodification, and internalized weight stigma requires a reclamation of our body as our home. We must take back that which has been stolen from us: the birthright to a body lived in with presence and delight. This beautiful book shows us how to remove the hooks that have kept us stuck and ashamed. Well done."

—Amy Pershing, LMSW, ACSW, CCTP-II, coauthor of *Binge Eating Disorder: The Journey to Recovery and Beyond*

"This book, and the Body Stories generously shared throughout it, are portals of possibility for a more compassionate, connected, and joyful relationship with your body, and a world where each of us knows the truth of the safety, dignity, and belonging that is our birthright."

—Nicola Haggett, body liberationist and certified Body Trust Provider

"With their trademark poetic style, Hilary and Dana hold us gently yet steadily, offering so many opportunities to reflect and explore difficult or even painful experiences with clarity, compassion, and courage as they guide us home to where we've always belonged—ourselves."

—Fiona Sutherland, founder of The Mindful Dietitian

"The journey towards embodiment can feel overwhelming—or even impossible— after growing up in a society that taught you to hate your body. *Reclaiming Body Trust* is a steady and compassionate hand that will support you while taking those first steps."

—Jes Baker, coach, speaker, and author of *Landwhale* and *Things No One Will Tell Fat Girls*

"Hilary and Dana outline how grace through Body Trust can help many achieve what they've always really wanted—to just feel good in their skin."

—Shelby Gordon, speaker, retired professional dieter, anti-racism consultant, diet-culture historian

"This book invites you into relationship with your own appetites and hungers. This book will nourish you and give you permission to seek pleasure and joy. Hilary and Dana will remind us of the messiness of this healing journey and remind us to do it imperfectly."

—Rachel Millner, PsyD, CED-S, CBTP, psychologist and eating-disorder specialist

"Hilary and Dana hold a steady presence at our backs as we begin to heal from the legacy of anti-fat bias that has been handed down to us—calling forward new ways of being with ourselves and each other. Stitching back and forth between experiences and their meaning, *Reclaiming Body Trust* helps us understand the politics of how we got here, then helps answer the question I am often asked as a therapist, 'What can I do?'"

—Carmen Cool, MA, LPC, CHT, psychotherapist

"*Reclaiming Body Trust* is a manifesto to the heart of every person who ever had to shrink on an airplane or who was put on Weight Watchers as a kid. May this book be a companion to you as you find your way back to yourself. This is a book for unlearning, reclaiming, and for liberation."

—Anna Chapman, founder of #fatselfcaretips

"Body Trust addresses the rupture so many of us have with our bodies as we navigate diet culture, oppression, illness, disability, and aging. Hilary and Dana bring together decades of experience and stories to provide a guidebook for this journey back to ourselves."

—Lisa Erlanger, MD, clinical professor emeritus of family medicine, University of Washington School of Medicine

"Hilary and Dana have written such a wholehearted and tender invitation to reconnect with our bodies. Full of wisdom and hope, this is a brave and radical book that also manages to be accessible and very human. Hilary and Dana hold the stories of our bodies with such care—this book is a gift to anyone who will read it."

—Vicky Bellman, MNCS-accredited, UK-based therapist

"Offering easy-to-digest unpacking of BS science and cultural values, realistic and grounded examples of rituals and practices for forward motion, and the diverse personal stories of community members, *Reclaiming Body Trust* is like having a pocket-sized body-liberation workshop you can carry with you. The reverberations of the impact of this book—and the transformation it offers—will be palpable."

—Melissa A. Fabello, PhD, author of *Appetite: Sex, Touch, and Desire in Women with Anorexia*

"If you've ever wondered why you struggle to trust your body, within these pages is your answer. If you've ever wondered how to come home to your body in a world that makes doing so very difficult, within these pages is your map."

—Rachel W. Cole, intuitive-eating counselor and life coach

"*Reclaiming Body Trust* will shake the foundation of the diet industry with its clarity, compassion, and galvanizing call that we stop warring with ourselves and instead learn the power of trusting our bodies. The care and expertise with which Dana Sturtevant and Hilary Kinavey invite us to return home to ourselves will resonate for generations."

—Dawn Serra, sex and relationship coach

Reclaiming
Body Trust

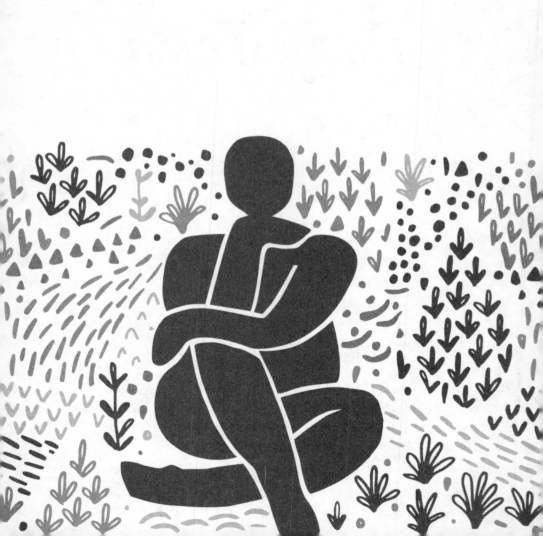

Reclaiming
Body Trust

A PATH TO HEALING
& LIBERATION

**Hilary Kinavey, MS, LPC,
and Dana Sturtevant, MS, RD**

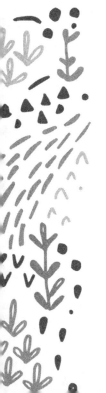

a TarcherPerigee book

tarcherperigee

an imprint of Penguin Random House LLC
penguinrandomhouse.com

Most TarcherPerigee books are available at special quantity discounts for bulk purchase for sales promotions, premiums, fund-raising, and educational needs. Special books or book excerpts also can be created to fit specific needs. For details, write: SpecialMarkets@penguinrandomhouse.com.

Grateful acknowledgment is made for permission to reprint the following: "I Woke Up Like That," by Angela Braxton-Johnson, © November 2017; originally published in *Unchaste Anthology*, vol. 2, Jenny Forrester, ed. (Portland, OR: Unchaste Press, 2017); "She Majestic Tree," by Angela Braxton-Johnson, © July 2018. Used by permission of the author; Excerpt from "Sangha," in *Go In and In: Poems from the Heart of Yoga* by Danna Faulds. (Berkeley: CA: Peaceable Kingdom Press, 2002). Used by permission of the author.

Library of Congress Cataloging-in-Publication Data
Names: Kinavey, Hilary, author. | Sturtevant, Dana, author.
Title: Reclaiming body trust: a path to healing & liberation /
Hilary Kinavey, MS, LPC, and Dana Sturtevant, MS, RD.
Description: [New York]: TarcherPerigee, [2022] | Includes index.
Identifiers: LCCN 2022017131 | ISBN 9780593418666 (hardcover) |
ISBN 9780593418673 (epub)
Subjects: LCSH: Body image. | Reducing diets—Social aspects.
Classification: LCC BF697.5.B63 K568 2022 |
DDC 306.4/613—dc23/eng/20220418
LC record available at https://lccn.loc.gov/2022017131

Printed in the United States of America
1st Printing

Book design by Shannon Nicole Plunkett

We dedicate this book to those whose body stories, pain, and lived experiences have been disregarded and disbelieved and to the people who have lost their lives due to systemic and interpersonal weight stigma.

We also dedicate this book to Kyan and Luca, and all children in the world for whom we wish to preserve body trust. May they always feel at home in, and have reverence for, their bodies.

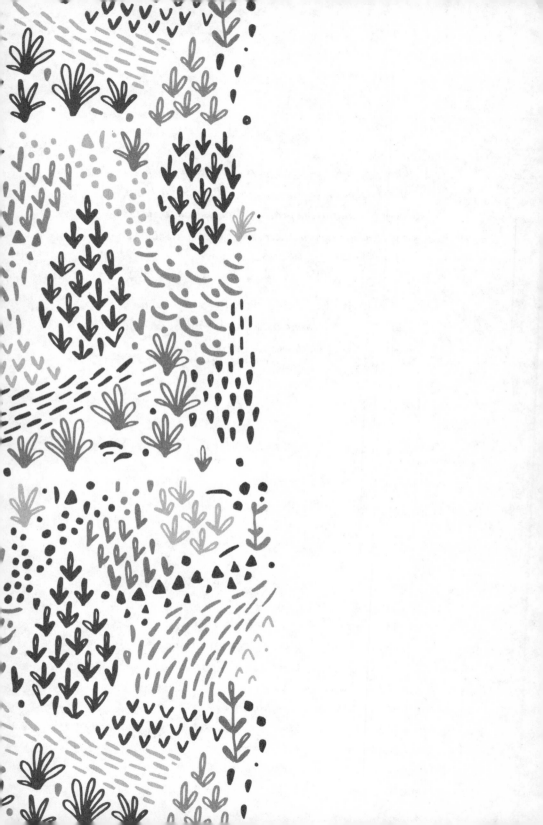

Contents

I Am a Person Reclaiming Body Trust

I am reclaiming trust in my body. My hunger, my appetites, my longings, my skin, my bones, my size are mine for the taking. I take back my voice, my agency, my worthiness, my belonging in the world of beautiful and diverse beings. I live without apology for the straight lines and curves, living tissue and vulnerable heart that hold my living, breathing manifested story.

I feel where my body begins, and I protect where it ends. The marketing, the expectations, the gaze of the "other" belong outside of me and are not for my internalization. I will no longer ingest the external and make it my goal or my standard. I will not trade my right to express my freedom, my dreams, my needs, my wants, or my beauty.

I listen for my appetites, all of them. I say yes. I say no. And I say not now. My body is wise. It knows me. It is me. I am it. My body is not an expression of gluttony or neglect, nor is it ugly. My body is an expression of life, and of being alive. It is my companion for this unfolding story, replete with unexpected bumps and grooves, loves and losses—and as such, my body expresses my story with its textures, rolls, shapes, peaks, and valleys.

I will not betray you, body, for an endless diet or self-improvement project. I will not confuse thinness for health. I will no longer objectify myself, nor will I continue to invest in oppressive beauty standards. I am a person reclaiming my movement, my rhythm, my flow. I seek satisfaction and explore pleasure. I value my inner peace, my self-worth, more than the approval of outside stigma and hate-inflicting eyes.

I will count myself among the millions of other people who have come before me in their struggles to live compassionately in the bodies they have, and I will also count myself among the millions to come who will reclaim their body and rebuild that trust. I am not alone on the path. In fact, I am helping to transition the world with my courage, my fierceness, my bold and beautiful body.

Introduction

What has come between you and feeling at home in your body?
How did you first come to learn that your body was a problem?

These are some of the first questions we ask people who attend our workshops, retreats, online courses, and professional training. If you've picked up this book, you've likely had a complicated relationship with your body. One that has led to years of body loathing and distrust, weighing and measuring, cycling through plan after restrictive plan, and feeling out of control and frustrated about food and your body.

You've likely tried a lot of different things along the way to feel in control. And the hustle created by this lifelong body project has left you feeling exhausted, angry, and unable to trust yourself.

You may notice how your tolerance to food restriction and dietary restraint has diminished over time. That the plans you were once able to follow for months, even years, now last a couple of days if you are lucky.

And any weight you may have lost on these plans has been regained, plus more.

You may feel at a loss for what to do next. You've tried so hard, for so long, and nothing seems to work.

You may not believe us when we tell you that none of this is your fault. You are not broken. We promise there doesn't need to be a separate set of rules for you.

But you may want to try something different instead of just trying harder.

Curious? If what we have shared so far is resonating, this book may be exactly what you need to get out of the endless cycle of shame and body blame.

The truth: Efforts to lose weight disconnect you from your body's wisdom. The $71 billion diet and weight loss industry thrives because nobody blames its plans when you can no longer sustain them. You blame yourself. You believe you have no willpower, that you can't be trusted with food, that you're addicted. So you return to these so-called experts to tell you what to do.

Here's another truth: These are experts in ideologies and a failed weight loss paradigm. There is no evidence-based treatment for weight that leads to sustained weight loss. A meta-analysis of twenty-nine studies on structured weight loss programs conducted in the United States found that participants regained 77 percent of their initial weight loss, on average, after five years.[1] No program has ever demonstrated long-term maintenance of weight loss for any but a small minority.[2,3]

We've basically all been duped. We've been socialized and indoctrinated into oppressive and mechanistic ways of thinking about the body before we are old enough to consent. Most people who have worked with us acknowledge they learned something was wrong with their body before the age of ten, many much earlier. As we age, we spend more time *thinking* about the body than *being* in the body. We believe the body must be tightly controlled, that thin equals healthy, that one meal or day of eating has the power to heal or kill us, and that all we have to do is get this "calories in versus out" equation right. It is an oppressive, inauthentic, and unsustainable way to occupy and care for a body.

The act of reclaiming body trust is both personal and political. We struggle, as a society, to understand the role discrimination, stigma, and oppression have played in the emotional and physical well-being of people with marginalized identities. We fail to see how our conversations about well-being have often bypassed the social determinants of health (poverty, trauma, environmental racism, genetics, etc.). We over-rely on personal responsibility and bootstrapping rhetoric (i.e., if you get sick, it's because you aren't living a "healthy lifestyle"). We often reinforce a hierarchy of bodies that is upheld across systems and institutions without questioning the validity of our knowing. An individual's worthiness is born from this, as well as the coping mechanisms that allow people to survive in a culture that doesn't truly value them. This book is about where and why that coping began, how it evolved, and how we begin to feel more free.

We are a therapist-dietitian team who cofounded the Center for Body Trust to help people heal from the effects of living in a weight- and health-obsessed world. We started our work together more than seventeen years ago after witnessing the harm caused by nutrition ideologies, toxic fitness culture,* and the traditional weight loss paradigm. We saw an urgent need to have different conversations with people about food, their bodies, their weight, their health, and their well-being.

Our Body Trust framework has evolved over time with our own learning and unlearning as two white, cisgender, currently able-bodied women who've had our own complicated relationships with our bodies. Because we cannot speak to all readers' lived experience, we have included stories and sourced the wisdom and expertise of others throughout this book to offer more perspectives. We've done our best, with the support and guidance from our teachers and mentors, to situate our work in liberatory frameworks and methodologies.

Body Trust is scientifically grounded and greatly informed by the following: Bobbie Harro's Cycle of Socialization and Cycle of Liberation; Barbara Love's Liberatory Consciousness; Desiree Adaway's Praxis of Liberation; Niva Piran's Developmental Theory of Embodiment (DTE); and Health at Every Size Principles; as well as intuitive eating principles, shame resilience theory, motivational interviewing,

---

* "Toxic fitness culture" is a term coined by Ilya Parker, founder of Decolonizing Fitness, https://decolonizingfitness.com/blogs/decolonizing-fitness/what-is-toxic-fitness-culture.

self-compassion theory, feminist therapies, mindfulness-based approaches, and postmodern therapeutic thought.

Dana has deep roots in the American Midwest and grew up solidly middle class in exurban Chicago. When she was sixteen, her family moved to Miami, Florida, and a whole new world opened in terms of culture and diversity. Dana has Norwegian and German heritage, is currently a size 16/18, and her body story includes weight teasing by high school friends, chronic pain, an autoimmune condition, and a four-year struggle with infertility. Dana completed both her bachelor's and master's degrees in nutrition science. Her training as a registered dietitian was steeped in the dominant weight paradigm, and ten years of her career was focused on helping people lose weight and keep it off (seven as a research interventionist and three as a bariatric dietitian). Like many health care providers, Dana believed she was promoting healthy lifestyles at the time, not dieting behaviors. As she became more skeptical of the advice she was giving and feared she was causing more harm than good, she discovered a growing community of helping professionals offering alternatives to the traditional ways she'd been trained to think about food, weight, and health. Feeling unethical in her work and knowing that any job in her field would expect her to help people lose weight prompted Dana to start a private practice, and this is where she met Hilary.

Hilary grew up in the San Francisco Bay Area surrounded by lots of loud and loyal Irish and Italian American family members who worked as tradespeople and helping professionals. She, and the people around her, lived with the impact of intergenerational mental health and addiction, which influenced her career path. She has lived in a small to mid-fat body throughout her life. She also lives with chronic health conditions. She came to this paradigm through her own ruptured relationship with her body that began with early dieting. This fork of her career path came unexpectedly, when, at the request of people she served, she began groups for people who had recently had weight loss surgery. In these groups, which offered an alternative conversation to the large group "which protein powder" conversations that dominated hospital-based support programs, she learned from participants about their true body stories, which countered the ones told through mainstream stories and therapeutic training. The lifelong nature of the appearance- and gender-based abuses they experienced, the complicity of previous mental and health care providers, and the challenge of navigating life as a fat person are some of the common themes that have permeated her practice for more than twenty years.

Over the years, we've listened to and been trusted with thousands of body stories from people with diverse identities and backgrounds, and we'll be sharing some of these stories with you in this book. Some were created from interviews. Others are personal narratives. Our hope is that you see parts of yourself reflected in these stories, as many are rarely truly heard and understood. We also asked Sand Chang, a genderfluid, nonbinary psychologist/Body Trust Provider, to write a letter about Body Trust for our trans and nonbinary readers. The following foundational beliefs have emerged from witnessing people's stories and shape everything in this book.

* We believe hypervigilance about food, fitness, weight, and health is harming people in significant and profound ways.

* We believe people are not required to pursue health in order to be deemed worthy of love, respect, and belonging.

* We believe nobody wins when we see a healthy body only as a thin one.

* We believe pleasure is a force essential to healing and liberation.

* We believe healing your relationship with food and your body is a vital part of feeling whole.

✳ We believe anti-fat bias, body oppression, and societal inequities make caring for your body difficult, and your suffering is not your fault.

We want you to know it is possible to have a better relationship with food and your body. We'd like to help you connect the dots between social justice and this healing work so you can begin to divest from diet culture, develop resilience to weight stigma and body shame, and return to the Body Trust we believe is your birthright.

So you might be wondering, What exactly is Body Trust?

Body Trust is a radically different way to occupy and care for your body. It is a pathway to reclaim your body and is completely counter to conventional "wisdom" about food, body image, weight, and health in our culture. Body Trust is . . .

✳ Getting out of your head and back into your body

✳ Deepening your analysis of what has come between you and feeling at home in your body

✳ Rejecting restriction and deprivation as a lifestyle or path to health

✳ Developing a relationship with yourself and your body that is flexible, compassionate, and connected

✳ Letting go of rigidity and perfectionism

✳ Grieving the illusion of control, the dream of being thin, the big reveal, the lost time/money/energy, the harm done, and more

✳ Turning toward your body, looking and listening with kindness and curiosity

✳ Stretching the outer edges of your body positivity until all bodies belong and are celebrated, including yours

*   Divesting from social constructs of beauty

*   Listening to your body and discerning the wisdom that comes from within

*   Allowing pleasure and satisfaction to finally inform and teach you, as much as what you know to be "good" or "healthy"

*   Knowing that when you eat past full or don't eat enough, your body's hunger cues can help guide you

*   Becoming attuned to your body's subtle and not-so-subtle cues

*   Acknowledging the incredible ways your body shows up for you every day

*   Moving your body in ways that feel revitalizing and connect you to sensation, pleasure, and joy

*   Rooting self-care practices in weight neutrality, and trusting your body to sort out the weight

*   Advocating for bodies with different access and privilege than your own

Now, it makes sense that you might be skeptical. We realize this book will challenge everything you've been taught to believe about weight, health, beauty, and worth. Pause for a moment and ask yourself: If my resistance to doing things another way could talk, what would it say?

This isn't going to work.

I can't trust this body.

If I listened to my body, I'd never stop eating _____.

I'm too broken.

Now ask yourself:

Who benefits from these beliefs?

Who is making money off your shame?

It's hard to be nourished in a culture that doesn't trust your body. When trust is lost in any relationship in your life, it takes time to get it back. When it comes to Body Trust, this trust is reciprocal— you are working on trusting your body and your body is working on trusting you. When you are restricting and restraining your food, your body doesn't know you are choosing not to eat. It thinks there must be a famine. If you are currently experiencing food insecurity or grew up with food insecurity, this adds another layer of complexity to your relationship with food. Regardless of the reason for a lack of consistent adequate intake, if/when food becomes available, your biological drive to eat kicks in in a desperate attempt to survive, and eating can feel "out of control." Imagine if you were stuck under water and deprived of oxygen for longer than your body could tolerate. When you finally made it above the surface, do you really think you'd just casually sip air to recover? *No.* You'd gasp for air in a panic until you got enough oxygen for your body to finally feel some relief. This frenzied feeling is about survival. There's a lot to unpack on the way to healing.

Before we talk about what you'll find in this book, let's be clear about what you *won't* find in these pages:

Weight loss promises: If we make promises about what will happen to your weight on your path to Body Trust, we are no different from anyone else you've sought to support you in this struggle. Your body has a weight where it's comfortable, and you can spend your whole life fighting to suppress it or you can move toward healing. In our seventeen-plus years doing this work, we've not found it possible for folks to heal the relationship with food (and body) while trying to control or change it,* which is why we encourage you to keep laying down your thoughts about weight and even health. We trust your body to sort out the weight.

"O" words: We will not be describing people's bodies using the words "obese" and "overweight" because these words, which are determined by using the body mass index, or BMI, are pathologizing, stigmatizing, and *not* evidence-based. Health is more complicated than a number on the scale, and being fat does not automatically mean one is unhealthy. In this book, you'll find more neutral descriptions of people's bodies, like larger-/smaller-bodied people, higher weight/lower weight people, and fat people. Now, we realize the word "fat" might not feel like a neutral descriptor, since it is weaponized against people. But there has been a movement since the 1960s (and likely before) to reclaim the word "fat" and strip it of its negative connotations. We use it the same way you'd describe a short body or a tall body. You can read more about the fat acceptance movement on our website.

Healthism: Upholding health as a moral imperative is harming people. This said, this book is not about health, it's about healing. Healthism is a set of beliefs that highlights health as the responsibility of the individual and ignores the influence of class, oppression, historical trauma, environmental racism, weight stigma, etc., on health. Healthism dissociates privilege from health status and relies on anti-fat bias and personal responsibility rhetoric, blame, and bootstrapping to promote health. In a paper entitled "Effecting Change in Public Health," Lucy Aphramor, PhD, RD,

---

* We are not talking about gender dysphoria and the life-affirming surgeries that lead to healing.

writes "lifestyle factors (health behaviours) account for as little as
5-25% of social differentiation in health outcomes . . . up to 95%
of inequalities in 'lifestyle diseases' can be explained by people's
experiences of oppression and trauma."[4] For those of you who have
spent a lifetime trying to control food and your bodies, shifting
the focus to healing your relationship with food and body not only
enhances your well-being but also helps you move on to something
more sustainable and supportive of your entire being. In our
experience, the preoccupation with improving "health" is really just
code to keep striving for food and body control and looks an awful
lot like an eating disorder. So we recommend saying "not now" to
thoughts about improving your health so you can focus on getting
untangled from all this and begin to root into something more
grounded and nourishing.

Nutrition advice: Most of the people we work with know way
too much about food and nutrition, and the last thing they need
is more dietary advice. Without adequate time to heal your
relationship with food, you'll find it hard to consider nutrition
without thinking about food and eating in binary ways like "good
or bad," "right or wrong," "healthy or unhealthy." Nutrition is
a relatively young field of study and what we read, watch, and
listen to on the subject is more of a philosophy or ideology than
a solid science. This book will distinctly center healing, which
in and of itself enhances health, as opposed to food and exercise
advice to improve "health." Many books about food and the body
are steeped in healthism (explained above) and nutritionism—a
reductionist way of thinking about food that assumes the
whole point of eating is to maintain and promote bodily health.
These ideologies can uphold an oppressive dieting mindset
and encourage people to strive for unnecessary, sometimes
harmful, and often unsustainable dietary practices. On the topic

of colonialism and nutritionism, Dr. Linda Alvarez, associate professor at California State University, Northridge, says,

> *Europeans believed specific foods shaped superior bodies. They introduced the idea of "you are what you eat." When they stepped foot on native land, they categorized indigenous foods as "bad" foods and European foods as "good" foods. They believed if they ate indigenous foods they would then turn native and therefore inferior. They went as far as banning certain plants for their medicinal and ceremonial use and rewarded "indios" for Europeanizing.*[5]

For now, we encourage you to put thoughts about nutrition, health, and weight on the back burner so you can begin to listen to your body instead of leading with your head. The personal food, eating, and self-care practices that emerge from your own truth will be much more supportive and sustainable in the long run.

Talk of food addiction: You may have heard that sugar lights up the same parts of the brain as heroin. This phenomenon is why many believe it is addictive. But you know what else lights up that part of the brain? Music, humor, a smile from a stranger, a good hug, and falling in love. But we don't seem to pathologize these things. Food addiction is a phrase that's been used in a wide variety of contexts, with increasing frequency over the past forty years to invoke many of the same ideas believed about drug addiction. New science finds, though, that many widely held beliefs about what we call addiction—to drugs, food, or many other things—are actually incorrect and harmful. We believe it is important that as society unlearns dangerous misconceptions about drug addiction that we not repeat the same mistakes in our efforts to help people have better relationships with food. We talk more about this in a later chapter.

Lots of talk about how to improve body image: Body image work doesn't quite cut it. It exclusively places the burden of healing upon the individual alone. We want systemic change and less body blame. The truth is, body image cannot sustainably improve without addressing the personal and systemic impact of anti-fat bias. The more deeply we are willing to dismantle institutions that monetize weight stigma, the more deeply people will be able to occupy their bodies. Internalized dominance and oppression and the resulting body shame have to be named not merely as "thinking errors," but as the very real experience of having a body that is subject to othering and pathologizing. Too many interventions focus solely on improving your body image. Body Trust is about turning toward and unraveling the body loathing, shame, dominance, and oppression that have turned your body into a thing needing to be altered and improved. This cultural stuff was never yours, though you may feel overrun by it. This book will help you question what you really want when you say you need to work on your body image. We want freedom for bodies and we want inclusion.

Scientific justification: Books evaluating the evidence for a shift toward weight-inclusive models of care like Body Trust have already been written (see Resources on our website). While science is important and will be included to some degree here, we also believe in other ways of knowing. We want to speak to the part of you that's been harmed by diet culture, anti-fat bias, and body-based oppression: the part of you that already knows the truth in the depths of your being.

Shortcuts: Reclaiming body trust is no small feat, so it makes sense you might be looking for a shortcut. Shortcuts and quick fixes are often how the diet, weight loss, and cosmetic fitness industries sell their snake oil. You might find yourself asking, "How do I cross the bridge from diet culture to body trust?" While we love this visual, there is important terrain to explore and discover that would be bypassed if we take the bridge instead of descending into the muck.

So much of what we desire to bring into our lives requires deep work before we can fully embody it. Body Trust is not a new plan, a gimmick, or a short-term solution, nor is it something you can rebuild simply by reading about it and understanding it intellectually. A heady exploration will get you only so far. To divest from diet culture and sink your roots more deeply into body trust, you will need to explore your body story, take risks, and work the edges of your comfort zone as you experiment with and practice the concepts in this book. And just like when you are learning any new skill, it will be awkward, bumpy, and clunky. It won't always be pretty. You may feel like you are flailing without the rigidity and rules of a plan. If you allow your inner critic to spin these challenges into a story about how you are "broken" and "you'll never get it right," you will abandon this work for a familiar program that helps you feel more contained from "the messiness." You may wander and then return. You will fall down and get back up. This is what it looks like in practice. Over time, it will get easier, we promise. There will come a time in your body trust practice where not doing it will be harder than doing it. For now, we want you to know body trust is not a place we arrive, but a connective energy we cultivate. It is an endeavor for a lifetime, and just as our bodies will not stay the same for a lifetime, our practice will shift and change to rise and meet our evolution.

Now, we realize after reading all this, you may be confusing Body Trust with something we like to call the "fuck it" plan. We assure you that **this is not the "fuck it" plan**. There's a lot of distance between the rigidity and perfectionism of a disordered, dieting mindset and the "fuck it" mentality. There's a big difference between letting go and giving up. Body Trust is more of a middle path . . . a place where we are not swinging from one extreme to the other. We live in the middle, away from binary thinking, in the land of discernment. It is realistic, it is sustainable, and it is internally sourced. It emphasizes your story and your truth by removing the middleman—the one who profits off trauma, stigma, and disembodiment.

As you can see by now, this is not your typical self-help book for food and body struggles. This book is an immersion into Body Trust and an invitation to bring a radically different healing paradigm into your life and into the world. It will offer you some time to think through all that diet culture has put you through. The information we share in these pages will help you better understand what the problem really is so you can break free from the status quo and reclaim and embrace your body. We delineate this path to healing in three phases: The Rupture, The Reckoning, and The Reclamation.

In the first part of this book—The Rupture—we'll begin to explore what it means to be embodied and help you understand how you lost trust with your body. We want you to know what we mean when we say Body Trust is your birthright. You were born with an inherent trust for your body, and somewhere along the way you became disconnected from this intimate way of knowing via trauma, oppression, illness, and social constructs of gender, race, sexuality, beauty, health, and weight. You'll explore your body story and begin to see your coping as a survival strategy rooted in wisdom.

In the next section—The Reckoning—we help you reckon with the ways your relationship with your body has been disrupted by harmful ideas, constructs, and practices in our culture. Body Trust requires you to come to terms with your humanity, your vulnerability, your own needs and desires, your genetics, your family history, your set point, and so much more. You will reckon with the ways you've been socialized, the lies you've been told, the harm that's happened, the years wasted, and the money and energy spent on the dream—and the illusion—of being in control. Body Trust asks you to make space for the grief that arises when you realize you've been duped and will never find what you've truly been looking for in another plan to control your food, your feelings, your body.

In the final section—The Reclamation—we describe the process of rebuilding trust with food, body, and self, and share how it is not all that different from how we rebuild trust in any relationship in our life when it is broken: through attunement and small consistent acts over time, not conditional acts or large-scale gestures.[6] Body Trust is a reclamation of your body, your voice, your story, and your own damn self. We'll explore the process of coming home, share ideas for reclaiming movement, and give you an opportunity to focus on finding joy and pleasure again, as you turn your attention toward the parts of you that perhaps you lost sight of in The Hustle.

This book is a part of and in service to a radical movement, and our work is preceded by fat activists, queer activists, and women of color who dared to say their bodies had value in a world that wanted only to pathologize, condemn, and silence them. By the time you are holding it in your hands, it is already a historical document. Language has likely evolved to be more inclusive, teachers we mention here have made mistakes or revealed more of their bias. We want to acknowledge there are teachers we quote in this book, because their work has been invaluable to the creation of Body Trust, who do not include fatness in their intersectional lens.* We've all been impacted by pervasive weight stigma in varying degrees and different ways. Our wish is that this book helps readers strengthen their liberatory consciousness to include all bodies so fewer people are colluding with the oppressive construct of diet culture.

We believe you can be transformed only by your own direct experience. This book, which is inquiry based, will reconnect you to your own

---

* "Intersectional" is a term coined by Kimberlé Crenshaw in "Demarginalizing the Intersection of Race and Sex: A Black Feminist Critique of Antidiscrimination Doctrine, Feminist Theory and Antiracist Policies," *University of Chicago Legal Forum* 1989, article 8 (1989): 139–67.

knowing, your deepest truths, and your inner wisdom. We hope it will meet you where you are and support the part of you that is in need of information and a new way forward. As coach Randi Buckley says, please consider context, nuance, and discernment to find what is true for you.[7] We've also created a web page with journaling prompts, supportive resources, and guided meditations to further assist you in the process of divesting from diet culture and deepening your roots into Body Trust. The deeper your roots, the stronger your practice.

There is a lot more to unlearn than there is to learn on the path to body trust. We encourage you to stay open, curious, and receptive, knowing that over time, more of these concepts will sink in. At the end of the book, you'll get to decide what you want to do with the information we share here. You may notice that you want body trust for everybody else, and still believe you need to change your body. This is a phase most of the folks we work with go through. Your process, your resistance, and your uncertainty are welcome here.

For now, we want you to know that we trust you, we trust your body, and we trust you with your body. We can hold that belief for you now. Our hope is that this book will help you hold it for yourself someday.

We believe this work is for every body. Every. Single. One. And that includes you.

We look forward to exploring with you.

Dana and Hilary

This book contains the stories of people's lived experience, struggle, and healing process. You will occasionally find specific depictions of weight loss strategies, some of which are also commonly exhibited in several eating disorders. We invite you to take care of yourself as you are reading and encourage you to ask for support when needed.

VICKY'S BODY STORY

I always loved the water, it's been a part of me since I was young. I used to go swimming as a kid. There was just the water and fun—no diet talk, no swim clubs, just swimming and enjoying. I've always been known as the person who will go into the sea, no matter the temperature. Even when I was five, six years old. I really liked that aspect of myself, that it was considered unusual. It really formed part of my identity.

When I was twenty-five, swimming became a part of my weight loss plans. I restricted food and really elevated my movement or exercise. It was really performative. I remember going to the swimming pool and feeling like I was one of them—the active people—with my gym bag. I had "the look" and felt like people would see me on the street with my wet hair and be able to say, Well, she's going to the gym and does so all the time. It was an athletic thing rather than a leisure thing, and that felt really good to me as a twenty-five-year-old, like an identity piece. An affirmation that became the whole point of swimming. I wasn't doing it for enjoyment whatsoever.

It was all about numbers. I counted each length, repeating the number to myself until the end and then repeating the next number. Over and over again. By the end I was doing a hundred lengths, four times a week. I was swimming the most extraordinary amount with no nourishment. I wanted so desperately to be seen as athletic. I didn't recognize that athletes need to nourish their bodies. To be clear, it was not really about athleticism. It was about weight loss. And I'm not sure I knew the distinction then.

It was about a look: slim and disciplined. It was also a really stealth way of having an eating disorder. It took me years to realize it was an eating disorder. No one said a thing, and I lost 55 percent of my body weight in eight months, which is painful to acknowledge. That would not fly under the radar of anyone in a smaller body.

My doctor was praising me for the weight loss. My GP knew I had a back specialist at the time but still praised me. They saw the weight dropping off me and it was nothing but praise.

My swimming was not the only thing that was very regimented. I would go to weigh myself once a week on the proper scales at the gym and intermittently through the week at home. I was also recording everything I was eating. I had little connection to my body.

As I was swimming I had no idea really what my body was doing. It was a machine, completely automated. 1, 1, 1, 1, 1, 2, 2, 2, 2, 2. There was no body connection. If my body had said anything then, I would've pushed. If I had had pain, I wouldn't have listened to it. My martial arts trainer at the time told me that "pain is weakness leaving the body." How can you say that with a straight face? He thought he was inspiring this fat little twenty-five-year-old. He thought he was gonna chisel me. Those words "pain is weakness leaving the body" played in my head when I was on lap 78 and my back started hurting, or I was bored. I'd push on. Pain is just weakness leaving the body. You are becoming stronger. You are more disciplined. You are not soft.

Now I can see how I was leaving my body. The intention was for softness to leave my body, but what actually happened is spiritual softness left my body. I really feel that it was just edges and lines and sequential numbers. When I say that now, I feel surprisingly anxious. It feels like a robbery . . . really violent.

I feel like I gave up my self. It was an intentional personal act, but it felt like it was culturally taken away from me. It was applauded. There was not a single person who said anything different. I would turn up to places with my own lunch in a Tupperware box. I'd have the same seven things for lunch every day for eleven months and it was just praised. Until the very, very end when someone said to me,

"But don't go too far." I had a glimpse of what I would now define as the narrow definition of my acceptable womanhood. When that person said that to me, I was, like, What? Hang on a second, you told me to do this. And now you want me to stop? "Not too much, though." It made me realize that if I had continued, I would have had to walk that precipice for the rest of my life.

At the time, I was also running three times a week on concrete, in crappy trainers. When I think back on it, I feel for my poor knees and back. I just think of everything being jarred by my movements. I had no idea how to run more safely because I'd had no experience of being taken seriously in terms of sports. Because my body was viewed as bigger in childhood, there had never been an encouragement of sports. So I didn't know I was supposed to have the right trainers, nor did I know there was a difference between running on concrete and running on grass.

All of this movement—the swimming, the running, and the martial arts—came to an end when I was running one day and my back completely went out. I had a car accident when I was younger. My back should be handled really delicately and I was just pounding, pounding, pounding. I think about those poor little shock absorbers in my back that had no juice in them. And they just gave out, my body gave up, and I was in bed for three months. I could barely move, all because of overtraining in a completely malnourished body. I will never run again. I just would not do that to my body. So I stopped doing all of the things and I put all the weight back on pretty quickly. I continued restricting, using the Whole30 program and the like (under the guise of health) for eighteen months. I wouldn't have said I was restricting.

When I was twenty-eight, I was thinking about a New Year's resolution, and I was about to do the same thing I did every January: have a month of healthy eating just to reset after the "extravagances" of Christmas. It felt like a balanced thing and I was doing it in a really nurturing way, but it was still rooted in restriction with a covert intentional weight loss goal. So I caught myself and thought, "How would it be if just one year we don't go into this making another New Year's resolution. How about if just for one year we try not restricting at all in any way, none of the good and bad foods, none of the dairy-free, you know, just no restriction at all and see how that is for a year. If it sucks, we'll go back." And then I never went back.

For fifteen years, I hadn't been to a gym. And when COVID-19 hit, I lost all accidental movement—running from the train and just walking around London. I was sitting online every day, seeing clients and my posture probably wasn't great. I could feel I was a bit hunched. One day, I was just sitting, and out of nowhere my body said, very clearly, you have to move me. And because I've been back in contact with my body for a long time, the only answer was to say okay. I could feel my chest open and a lot of positive, playful, childlike energy. I went to the ocean the next day. I just stretched out in the water. My body was really craving a chance to fully take up all of the reach of my body.

Now, when I describe swimming, it's a really spiritual thing. Like a baptism every time I get in the sea. What turned me toward the pool was other people and culture. What turned me to the sea was my history with the sea. What brought me back to the ocean was my body itself.

I am so glad I was listening, and able to hear it. How many cues did I miss when I thought my body was lazy because it was fat? When I was doing movement as a punitive thing, I was just telling my body what to do, at the same time being completely cut off at the neck. What did I miss?

In the ocean my healing process came together in an extraordinary way. Swimming now gives me the opportunity to connect with the sea, connect with my body, and take what the sea is offering me. I have to listen to the sea as much as I listen to my body because listening keeps me safe. My body gives me all of my data and then the sea gives me hers. If she says, you can't swim today, I don't, I wouldn't want any more power over the sea than I would my own body.

The ocean is so good at safeguarding the movement for me. Numbers don't exist in the ocean. I swam for ten months before I allowed myself to get a tracker. It felt important to not track because I wanted to explore the capacity of my body rather than do what a tracker tells me to do. When I use the tracker, I do as much as my body wants. I swim down the coast and back and then I come out and I'm interested to see what happened, data-wise. A quick check and that's that.

My experience in the ocean is liminal. It is the edge space. I'm so aware of my edges when I'm in the water, aware of every inch of my body boundary. I'm almost aware of everything my body is doing inside and out. I am more aware of my heartbeat. I'm more aware of how my limbs are feeling, and where they are. I know exactly where all the parts of me are. I'm aware of the coastline and feeling far away from everyone, but also completely connected to everything. Everything's restored to me within me, around me, because it's that universal experience.

When you have tasted that freedom and have that boundary for yourself to explore the trust, I don't know how I would walk back through that old door now. I don't know what would have to happen for me to stop trusting my body because I hold my body in such high regard now.

I don't think I would ever be able to abandon my body the way I did all those years ago. It's a really formidable force when you team up with your body. It's about restoring the trust that made me safe to my body again. Restoring that trust within my body keeps me safe in the water because I have access to all the information. Maybe we don't talk about that enough. We want our bodies to be restored to us, but actually our bodies need time to be restored to us too.

Deeping Your Roots into Body Trust®

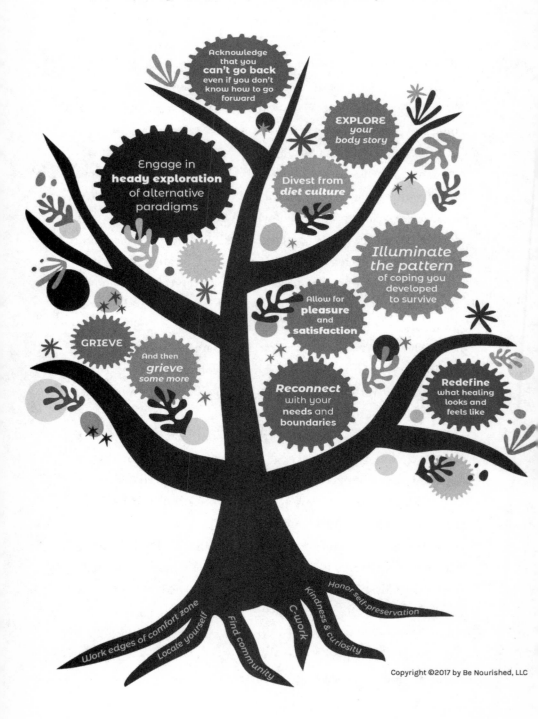

The Foundations of Body Trust

We use an image of a tree with roots to illustrate the ongoing and evolving process of reclaiming body trust. When you are new to these ideas and the seeds are just being planted, the concepts in this book need time to germinate and take root. In the meantime, because we are all socialized to have roots in oppressive ideologies that keep us fragmented and constantly striving, you will also be divesting—digging up the old roots. Many of us have a long and winding history in diet culture and anti-fat bias to root out.

Instead of telling you this should be easy if you put your mind to it, we want to let you know this work can be hard, but a different kind of hard than what you have internalized from diet and wellness culture. Body Trust work lives among ideas and practices that are different from mainstream culture and hard to accept. It is possible many people in your life are not going to get it.

This work is hard because it means uprooting the truth about what ruptured your relationship with your body, reckoning with the process of reclamation itself, and choosing to live a life where you do not participate in what has harmed you and which most of the culture deems benign. Embodiment coach and therapist Prentis Hemphill offers this truth: "When we are so shaped by the world that we are in, it only gets unmade through the risks we are able to take and by the risks we are willing to take. It unravels, in part, through risk. We have to be in relationship with risk. What risks will I take to unravel it? What risks will I take to be authentic? To be as alive as I can be?"[1]

The risk involved in considering change is often what sends us down paths of trying everything but the scariest thing. And the scariest thing might be giving up The Hustle—the cycle of trying to perfect food and change your body in the ways the world expects—to turn toward something more radically true that invites your whole being forward.

The truest thing about the unlearning process that is Body Trust is how we are never done. This, of course, is also the greatest challenge and frustration, especially in a culture of quick fixes, protocols, and externally derived definitions of recovery and success that tend to ignore the social inequities that make our lives not an "outcome" but an ongoing cycle of protecting and becoming.

The path to healing and liberation is multifaceted and nonlinear in part because you are doing this work in a toxic atmosphere filled with anti-fat bias, racism, transphobia, ableism, homophobia, ageism, misogyny, patriarchy, and white supremacy. Working with the various concepts, ideas, tools, and practices in this image will help deepen your roots into body trust. The deeper your roots, the more resilient you are when triggered or activated by the weather in the atmosphere. The shallower your roots, the easier it is for challenging (stormier) days to sweep you up and away and back on a familiar program or plan.

Over the course of the book, we'll share more about our Body Trust framework. First, we want to talk about the Foundations of Body Trust. Located in the roots of the tree image, these six foundations are essentially a pocketful of touchstones to help you let go of perfectionism and striving, return to your innermost work, and remind you of your humanity and your truest path—loving yourself and clearing the way for all bodies to have what they need to live their truth.

The foundations provide mooring. They ground you increasingly more deeply in the work and remind you of how the healing is in the return—to ourselves, our bodies, our truth. Healing comes through returning again and again, no matter how many times you feel lost or off course.

Work the Edges of Your Comfort Zone

We are more likely to grow and change when we are experiencing some discomfort. You don't have to go way out of your comfort zone to do this work, especially if you are just getting started. But we do our best learning, growing, and capacity building on the edges of our comfort zone. In fact, this is often where the magic happens . . . damn it!

It is normal to experience fear when we begin exploring Body Trust, in part because we have been socialized not to trust ourselves. Fear is not always a stop sign, though. It is sometimes a sign we are getting closer to the truth. We learned from Tara Mohr, author of *Playing Big: Find Your Voice, Your Mission, Your Message,* about how the Hebrew language has two words for fear: pachad and yirah. Pachad is the fear we experience when there is the threat of danger (fight, flight, freeze). Yirah is the fear we have when we are about to take up more space than we are comfortable with. When you experience this kind of fear, we encourage you to stay curious so you don't miss out on the wild, transformative part. Allow for some of the discomfort to arise without turning away from it.

When you are feeling unsteady, look for core beliefs, narratives, or fears telling you that you cannot change. These, though often unpleasant in tone, ground us in our comfort zones where we are less likely to change in the ways we so deeply desire. Your inner critic gets loud when you are about to take an important step. Tara Mohr writes, "it is like a guard at the edge of your comfort zone."[2]

We encourage you to create opportunities to work at and stretch the edges of your comfort zone, not go way outside of it—the point at which you experience hyperarousal, which may include anxiety, fear, panic, defensiveness, and/or hypervigilance. This is a state of flight or fight where you may also notice your mind ruminating, or you feel stuck on certain ideas of right or wrong. Or you may experience hypoarousal, which is characterized more by numbness, little access to emotion, low energy, and a lack of interest or motivation. It might be particularly hard to know what you are feeling, what you need and want.

Naming, honoring, and acknowledging the coping skills that have arisen from shame, guilt, and patterns of self-harm can, over time, change the way you respond to inner cues. We cannot change the world immediately. We do not want to gaslight or control our own coping in reaction to cultural and systemic harm. We do not need to earn our own love or self-reverence. The truth of our experience will move us forward. Your presence is not a burden, nor is it your fault that sometimes it's too much to bear.

Work those edges by sometimes doing the hard thing. Give yourself permission to eat what you really want. Have the difficult conversation, say no, honor your truth no matter how inconvenient. Move through all your stages of consciousness with acceptance, knowing they have protected you and will continue to until they are no longer needed.

Learning new things takes practice. It's not going to go as well as you may need it to at first because it is new. With some regular, consistent practice, there will come a time when not doing it will be harder than doing it. Just keep returning, over and over again. You can be trusted.

Look with Kindness & Curiosity

One thing we know for sure is that if beating yourself up and talking to yourself like you are a horrible human being worked, you would have arrived a long time ago! Wisdom and guidance rarely follow when we are full of contempt for ourselves. Kindness and curiosity are the opposite of the tough love, "power through it" ideals that typically prevail in wellness and diet culture. As you begin this work, we encourage you to move away from negative stories about you and your body that you tell yourself and instead tell yourself the kindest narrative possible.

There are lots of misconceptions about self-compassion. Many people believe they will simply throw in the towel if they are gentler with themselves. Or they will end up in a place of passivity or not caring. What we are actually talking about here is not giving up, but rather, letting go (more on this in chapter 6, "What Does Grief Have to Do with It?"). Research from Kristin Neff, one of the world's leading experts on self-compassion, actually shows how self-compassion is associated with more intrinsic motivation, learning and growth goals, curiosity and exploration, and less fear of failure.[3]

There is a difference between tough love and holding yourself gently accountable. There is a difference between how integrity and brute force look and feel. Love is a verb, yes? An action. So we keep at it. Feeling in alignment and in integrity with yourself creates the conditions for a solid place to land when you mess up. A gentle place. A real place. Meeting yourself in your humanity is the work.

One phenomenon we have noticed about most people who come to this work is how they want body acceptance, affirmation, and fat liberation for everyone but themselves. They want the world to be accepting and to believe body stories. They want people to have access to more peace and to the truest expression of themselves. And then they get stuck: *Why am I included? Why do I deserve peace? Can I opt for safety in the fucked-up but familiar instead of stretching into more discomfort?* Maybe not. Maybe this is exactly why you are here. To allow for change. To trust growth and to let things become different.

Practicing this stuff is not sexy at all. It is hard work and it is not fun, but it will have long-term payoff. Tara Brach, a Buddhist teacher and the author of *Radical Acceptance*, came up with an acronym, RAIN, to help people be kinder to themselves when big feelings and life's intensity threaten to pull us into disembodied coping:

Recognize what is happening;

Allow the experience to be there, just as it is;

Investigate with interest and care;

Nurture self-compassion.[4]

A key component of self-compassion is talking to yourself with kindness, the way you would if the same thing were happening to a beloved friend. This can be hard after a lifetime of feeling shame, self-blame, and listening to your own very intense inner critic. Some people tap into a gentler, more compassionate voice by placing their hand on their heart. Others think about what a loved one would say to them right now if they could see their suffering. Phrases like, "Oh, sweetie, it's okay" or "You did the best you could with what you had in the moment." Body Trust participant Maya G. told us,

> Self-compassion was exactly what I needed to tie all of the pieces together. This work of being human is not easy, and it's even harder when you hate the one person who will always be there. I decided to be kind, compassionate, and loving toward myself, and it makes everything else easier.

Here's one more thing to hold on to: the way you talk to yourself impacts your health and well-being, just as much if not more than doing whatever it is that makes you feel so full of self-loathing. View yourself with kindness and curiosity, and you will be surprised to see what becomes possible in this healing work.

Go for a C- (as Opposed to an A)

When we tell people to go for a C- in this work (as opposed to an A), they are often surprised—and a little resistant—only to later find this to be one of the most helpful foundations for deepening their roots into body trust. Diet culture and perfectionism go hand in hand. This work is messy, uncertain, different, imperfect, and human. We encourage doing this kind of badly some of the time (but not all the time), and remembering how this will get easier with time and practice, not in relentlessly chasing perfection.

Perfectionism tends to use us by keeping us compliant and always hustling. It has a way of upholding objectification and thus dehumanizing us. Your inner critic upholds this within you, often increasing demands when you most urgently need to be compassionately seen and understood. Start by noticing when perfectionism shows up in your life regarding food and your body. Come up with one sentence or phrase you can say to your critical voice to give you more space, like *I'm not doing that right now* or *Cut the shit.*

It's common for people to feel like they are flailing when they start on their path to body trust. When you go on another diet or new plan, you know within minutes or hours if you are "doing it right." This work isn't like that. When we are learning (or relearning) a skill, behavior, or practice, it takes time. We fall down and get back up. We learn as we go and grow, change, and practice.

When you begin to embrace the concept of C- work, experimenting and taking risks becomes more possible. It's easier to approach eating with the attitude of just seeing what happens when we do this versus that. With the concern of "getting it right" reduced, there's more permission to try new things.

Locate Yourself & Widen the Lens

As you do this work, we encourage you to widen your lens and locate yourself in the broader landscape. The rampant anti-fat bias in our culture impacts all of us, but it is not impacting us all in the same way. We all have dominant and nondominant identities and differing access to healing work. Your path will be unique because of your intersecting identities and where you are on any given spectrum. Understanding your social location can help you recognize your privilege, externalize the ways body blame and oppression have harmed you, and position yourself to center the ultimate purpose of this work: to create conditions for all bodies to be free. We must learn to own who we are in this conversation. We often ask the people we work with to "locate yourself." You can ask yourself: What am I bringing to this? What would change if I did a YOU-turn and saw myself through the eyes of others with less privilege and power?

A key touchstone in this work is continuing to locate the problem outside of our bodies. When you remember how we are all socialized and indoctrinated into harmful ways of thinking about and inhabiting a body, it becomes easier to recognize how patriarchy, white supremacy, and capitalism inform the way we view ourselves and others.

"Locating yourself" can also mean anchoring yourself in the present moment. Many of us have experienced moving through the world like a floating head, completely wrapped up in *our thinking mind*, disconnected from experiences below the neck. We recommend building up a regular, consistent practice of checking in with yourself and noticing where you are, what and who are in the room with you, naming colors and objects you see, being aware of your butt in the chair. Taking time to connect to the present moment and get below the neck offers new information for navigating your life. Start by pausing now, close your eyes, place a hand on your heart, and ask yourself a few of these questions, *How am I doing? How is it in there? How is my heart? How is my nervous system? What's my body need from me right now? Has my head/mind been dominating my experience with shitty, ruminating thoughts? Am I believing everything it says? Can I remember what else might be possible? Where am I physically and emotionally in this moment? What's happening and what do I specifically need?* Tending to yourself in this way even just once a day can begin to create a shift in awareness. And choice happens when we pay attention.

Lastly, when we get triggered and want to feel in control of food, our bodies, our emotions, and our lives, we often zoom in on a solution (restrained eating and compensatory exercise) that can fix the so-called problem, thinking everything will be better when we just "get it right." When we do this work, we begin to notice the tendency to zoom in and resist it by "keeping the lens wide" and looking at the entirety of our lives and all that being human brings with it—complications and messiness.

Find Community & Share Your Process

There are many people in our lives who are not ready to support anti-diet ideas, Body Trust work, and fat liberation, so we need to know there are other people on this healing path and find opportunities to connect with them. Support often precedes change.

Experiencing an equitable community is where healing becomes more possible. It may be helpful to spend a moment thinking about whether you have been in a community that is united around change and shared liberation. Bobbie Harro, the creator of the Cycle of Liberation and the Cycle of Socialization, says that uniting with a community of people who've chosen to interrupt the cycle of socialization and fight for change can bring "a sense of hope and optimism that we can dismantle oppression. They share a sense of their own efficacy—that they can make a difference in the world. They empower themselves and they support each other. They share an authentic human connection across their differences rather than fear because of their differences. They are humanized through action; not dehumanized by oppression. They listen to one another. They take one another's perspectives. They learn to love and trust each other. This is how the world changes."[5]

A Fat Babe Pool Party has become one space that has fortified many and cemented the essentialism of being in a fat-positive community. People throughout the movement have talked about how liberating it was to attend their first Fat Babe Pool Party, and the experience was re-created by writer Samantha Irby in season 1, episode 4—"Pool"—of the Hulu series *Shrill*. Aidy Bryant's character, Annie, cautiously shows up to the pool party, expecting to feel safer keeping her clothes on, initially finding difficulty in imagining that she would see herself in the fat babes around her. In her TED talk, fat activist Virgie Tovar said this about her experience:

> I saw something that I'd never seen, something I had been told did not exist. All around the pool were gorgeous fat women in amazing bathing suits. They were laughing and chatting, they were swimming and napping, they were just living without any discernible trace of the shame . . . I saw the potential for my own shame-free future.[6]

We developed our Body Trust framework sitting with groups of people who desired a different relationship with food and their bodies, and we've witnessed the efficacy of exploring this work in fat-positive spaces. Lauren, a Body Trust Provider in Edmonton, Alberta, says,

> When I was doing the Body Trust training, it was the first time I had been in a room full of people that I knew weren't judging me, and when we ate lunch, I remember there being a specific lunch, and I was able to just eat without qualifying. I didn't have to make excuses about the fact that I was hungry and wanted more. I was able to talk openly about how delicious it was and how much pleasure I was getting from food. That was really the first time that I had ever experienced that kind of freedom. It was life-transforming.

Your healing process will benefit greatly from finding *at least* one other person to share this journey with who won't gaslight you. If you struggle to find community, check out our website for ideas and a directory of Body Trust Providers who've trained with us, and consider curating a social media feed with messages that reinforce this work. There are lots of fat affirming, anti-diet accounts out there.

When you, your body story, and your efforts to heal are seen and heard, your roots in this practice will deepen. When in doubt, remember there is a growing community of people shouldering you in this work.

Honor Your Self-Preservation Practices

Honoring the ways we have survived is sometimes how we understand the depth of our own experience and wisdom. When you are in a storm, feeling lost or unmoored, or far away from Body Trust work, we urge you to return to the practices that have preserved and supported you. Sometimes self-preservation means we take comfort in what's familiar and available. Sometimes self-preservation means we set more boundaries, we allow ourselves to take time with decisions, and we center reverence for ourselves and our process.

Why self-preservation and not self-care? Self-care is often more performative than meaningful because of the ways the wellness industry co-opts and packages it for privileged people. Deeply nourishing practices bring us home to ourselves. They don't make us look to so-called experts to tell us how to live.

Coming home to ourselves when we have been conditioned to ignore and abandon our own knowing is going to take some time. We are not used to checking in with ourselves, asking questions about what we really want . . . or need, noticing if we like what we are eating or if how we are spending our time nourishes our well-being. So as you embark on this journey with us, give yourself some grace. You will at times lean on old coping behaviors that you consider maladaptive and don't always honor your full or evolving self.

We believe some of the magic in this work is in the owning of the utility and wisdom of your self-preservation practices. Self-preservation is how we keep going even when we don't want to. It is connected to what we believe is the reason we are here and alive. Self-preservation might be letting go of trying too hard and going for C- work. Self-preservation might mean putting aside fear or insecurity to take a risk to connect with others, despite what the hurt voices within are screaming at us. Self-preservation may also be taking a step back, using a way of coping that you wish you had never met and then moving on. Sometimes self-preservation is sourced from the light and sometimes it is from the familiarity of the shadows.

What does self-preservation look like for you? Start to make yourself a long, generous list of all the practices that make you feel rooted, grounded, connected, and whole. If this is hard, that's important information to know. Be gentle with yourself and consider returning to this question after reading more of this book. After making your list, highlight a few that are calling to you and set an intention to begin exploring them. Maybe put them on a Post-it and place it somewhere as a reminder to practice. Human beings are easily distracted by the busyness of life and get swept up in the familiar habits of the day. Gentle reminders are helpful when we want to practice new ways of being. Think progress, not perfection. C- work!

We understand that if you are new to this conversation, or you're diving deeper into your healing process, it may feel as though you are proceeding into something amorphous, so different from how it felt when you have started other programs. We want these six Body Trust foundations to feel like touchstones in your pocket or bumpers in your bowling gutter. Diet culture has conditioned us to give up, to believe we will either muscle through or fail. In truth—to keep going—we just go it slow sometimes and we call in an assist. These foundations may serve to bring you back to center, to widen your lens just enough to continue to turn toward feeling, believing in something different instead of cycling with something harder.

Choose one or two foundations that feel accessible and resonate with you. Write them on a stone and slide it in your pocket so they are available when you feel compressed, lost, scared, or worried. Or scribble on a Post-it Note that you stick to your phone so you can rely on them daily or lean on them in a storm. Make the foundation your practice and see what happens. No pressure. C- work. You deserve something different.

Part I

The Rupture

The act of reclaiming body trust involves acknowledgment of where your ideas about your value and worth have roots in the culture. How body trust was ruptured is not always immediately evident to us. In fact, we often internalize the idea that our body is a problem that we created, and therefore we are responsible for resolving it. The first section of the book is an invitation to think about how your relationship with your body has evolved. What we know—and want you to know—is that what has happened has not been your fault. There is no repentance necessary. Your coping has been rooted in wisdom, and we aren't here to take away anything you need to survive. What we wish to do is pull back the veil on ideas that have blamed you and made the size of your body the problem. We want you to have clear sight on all that has come between you and being at home in your body. There's often a strong sense of urgency to get it all resolved, but moving forward too fast can obscure the truth of your lived experience. So first, we create some space for the emergence of your truest story.

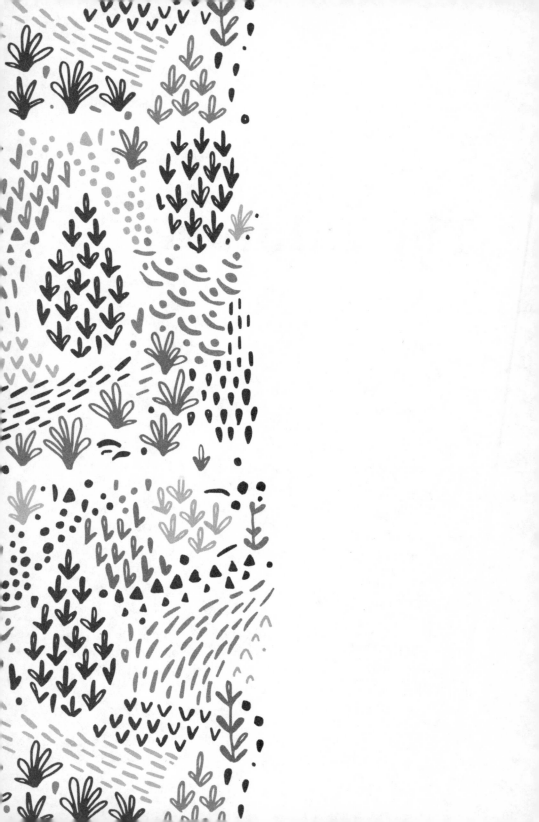

CHAPTER 1

Body Trust
Is a Birthright

We are easier to control when parts of
ourselves are fragmented.

—DESIREE ADAWAY

When we are born into this world, most of us feel at home in—and trust—our bodies. We do not fret about the size of our bellies, butts, or thighs, try to control our feelings, or worry about how the food we eat will impact our bodies. When we are born into this world, we are not aware of gender norms or racism, of what being trans or gay means. When we are born into this world, we are expressive beings, taking up space in unapologetic ways. We embrace our bellies and dance like nobody's watching. We put on clothes and don't worry about what people will think. We attempt to communicate with the adults in our lives when we have unmet needs: crying when we are hungry or dissatisfied, screaming when we really want to be heard. When we are born into this world, we are clear about what we like and we have no problem letting others know when we do not like something. We don't worry about being "too much" or "not enough." We are connected to our own knowing. We just are who we are.

For many, this oneness with our bodies lasted a very short time, and for others it slowly changed with age. So, what changes? As we grow, our socialization begins, the earliest seeds being planted at home with the people we love and trust. We are exposed to the ways the culture and the people around us categorize whose bodies matter and whose don't. We overhear diet talk at the table, along with Grandpa's disparaging comments about fat people. We watch Mom get dressed and say nasty things about her body. Fatphobia and the obsession with controlling food, weight, and/or health is often passed down from one generation to the next, sometimes as a form of protection from being "othered." Here's what a few Body Trust participants shared with us:

Nicole K. was seven years old when she first learned something was wrong with her body. She says, "I had tried on my new dance costume for the upcoming recital and was so excited to show my mom. As I entered the room, she said something like, 'Oh, Nicole, your stomach . . .'" I was puzzled. What? What about my stomach? I examined myself in the mirror and noticed an ever-so-slight curvature beneath the waistband of my hot pink spandex pants. Is that what she was talking about? And there, in that instant, a seed of self-doubt was planted."

Kari writes: "Historically, women in my family were most valued by their appearance, and by that I mean how thin they were. 'Boys get the pancakes, girls get the cornflakes' (Kellogg's Special K) for breakfast was the rhyming phrase which sang in tune with the constant litany of internal self-hate messages which I first remember around eleven years old. I had a childhood illness that was only made better by enormous doses of steroids. This resulted in extreme weight gain and brought me to my first Weight Watchers meeting at the age of twelve. Looking back, my starting weight on the program would be in the midrange of my 'goal weight' by today's standards."

In addition to listening to the adults around us, children's TV shows, and movies reinforce gender roles and racist beauty standards, with "good" thin characters (usually white) and "bad" fat characters (often "ugly" and non-white). And all the while, we are unconsciously conforming to these views.

We are all embodied into social systems that hold power. We live at these complex intersections of size, class, race, ethnicity, citizenship status, religion, age, gender identity, ability, and sexuality; and these identities impact the ways we engage with the world and our ability to feel at home in our bodies. Our bodies exist in systems that value and legitimize certain presentations over others, and this fuels and feeds research and popular opinion. Bobbie Harro, who developed The Cycle of Socialization, says, "We have been exposed, without initial question, to a strong set of rules, roles, and assumptions that cannot help but shape our sense of ourselves and the world."[1] Take a moment to think about these questions about your earliest socialization:

* What are some of your earliest memories of having a body?

* How did you first come to learn that certain bodies were better than others?

* What early messages did you receive about "other" people?

* What are some childhood experiences that impacted your ability to feel at home in your body?

* Write down at least five examples of what you learned it means to be fat.

* How were the seeds first planted that "being fat is bad"?

In her body story, Angela Braxton-Johnson, Body Trust Coach and founder of Poetically Inspiring Change, writes:

When did the Rupture of my body trust happen?

Well, let's just start with the harsh fact that I was born into a country where White Supremacy set the tone for just about everything, even much in the Black community. A construct that denied my cute little Black, fat body equality and acceptance right from jump street. So yeah, there's that.

Then add to that a long string of traumatic occurrences that aided in the breaking of my body trust.

Though I don't have a mental memory of some of those things, like being born into a home where domestic violence happened, I know that my body remembers.

Huge fractures in my body trust were caused by me being separated from my family when Mama moved us to the Pacific Northwest for a fresh start. A city where we had only one blood relative. Being transplanted from the very diverse DMV area (DC/Maryland/Virginia) to the very white state of Oregon was a culture shock for both Mama and me. Being sexually and physically abused at ages three and four. Being teased on playgrounds and parks, from the East Coast (during summer visits) to the West, from preschool to high school, just for being fat, which is part of being me. Being sexually abused by an older boy. Being bullied during first and second grades by some really mean girls. All of these experiences conveyed to me that I was very broken and not as worthy as kids who weren't fat.

Our earliest socialization in a weight-obsessed world is reinforced when we go to school, attend church, play sports, dance, etc. We receive consistent messaging from doctors, our after-school providers, the social workers, and food assistance programs, so it is no surprise that we do not question what we are learning. Diet culture is a combination of language, patterns of thought, beliefs, and practices reinforced by the media, medicine, academia, and popular culture. It is in the atmosphere in which we live and breathe. Diet culture is embedded in neoliberal ideas such as personal responsibility rhetoric, bootstrapping, healthism, and beauty standards, and then filters itself through clever marketing, fear mongering about size, and fatphobia disguised as care. It's quite a successful racket.

You may be finding yourself thinking about whether what we say is true for you and reflects your experience. Consider a few of these questions:

* What did you learn about bodies in school? In health class?

* How did your experiences with physical education (in gym class) affect your relationship with your body?

* What shows did you watch? How diverse were the bodies? What messages were reinforced?

* What did the adults in your life teach you about weight and health?

* Who encouraged you to count calories, weigh yourself, exercise to burn calories?

* How and where did you learn to think about food as good/ bad, right/wrong, healthy/unhealthy?

While we are socialized in a culture of body hierarchies, where there is always something better to strive for, we are also indoctrinated into a rigid, mechanistic way of relating to and managing the "unruly" body and all the ways our bodies don't necessarily do what those in power say they are supposed to do. In an interview for Roxane Gay's month-long anthology "Unruly Bodies" with Medium on what it means to live in a human body today, Kiese Laymon says:

> *I could make the argument that all bodies are unruly. I think that we do a lot to police the kinds of bodies that stick out of the norm. We don't like to talk about the violence we do to those bodies that, on the surface, are not supposedly nor-*

mal, which in this culture means cis, hetero, white, and thin.
There's obviously violence inherent in a culture which makes
particular kinds of bodies seem unruly.[2]

What most of us have been commonly taught about bodies is either a lie or a very narrow truth. Bodies are not all thin and some never will be. Not all bodies are healthy and some never will be. They are not all capable of athleticism or having boundless energy. That should not signal that people are doing something wrong or that they are not living happy, fulfilling lives. We learn to feel shame about our bodies, to worry about food, to lean into control and avoid feeling vulnerable, to avoid having an unruly body. And in doing so we ignore that health is most impacted by societal, environmental, and genetic elements outside of our immediate control.

Puberty is an especially ripe time for the beginning of a disrupted relationship with food and the body (if people are lucky enough to make it that far!). The natural weight gain at the onset of puberty is when many people and/or their parents get concerned. We are not taught to trust our body, that this weight gain is actually necessary for the hormonal changes our bodies are going through. We are not told to stay calm and let the body do what it needs to do, that we can trust the body to sort it all out. (This is also true for the natural weight gain that occurs later in life as we move toward our senior years and need weight to protect our bones and give our body the reserves needed if/when we get sick.)

Research has shown that for people who menstruate, the entry into and exit from reproductive life are the highest risk times for the development of an eating disorder. For transgender folks, the body changes that come with the hormonal shifts of puberty may kick off or amplify the experience of gender dysphoria and restrictive food and/or compulsive exercise patterns emerge to attempt to control and shape the body and attain oppressive gender norms. Longtime activist Suzanne Pharr writes: "It is at puberty that the full force of society's pressure to conform is brought to bear. Children know what we have taught them, and we have given clear messages that those who deviate from standard expectations are to be made to get back in line. The best controlling tactic at puberty is to be treated as an outsider, to be ostracized at a time when it feels most vital to be accepted. Those who are different must be made to suffer loss."[3]

It's no wonder that by the time we are teenagers, so many of us have a ruptured relationship with our body and end up adopting "the body project"—or as we refer to it in this book, The Hustle. As we age, we spend more time thinking about the body (objectifying it) than being in the body (subjectively experiencing it "below the neck"). We are made to believe the body must be tightly controlled, that thin equals healthy, that one meal or day of eating has the power to heal or kill us, and that all we have to do is get this "calories in/calories out" equation right. It is an inauthentic and unsustainable way to occupy a body and violates the body trust we believe is a birthright.

A physician, who preferred to remain anonymous, shared some of their body story with us:

> I was always a fat kid. I grew up in a family where fat was absolutely unacceptable so I was taken to a lot of doctors who told me miscellaneous things about my body, what it meant to be fat and how to stop being fat.
>
> Any encounter I had in the medical field growing up was traumatic. And I'm still traumatized by the medical field. One of the ways I decided to process that trauma was by diving in headfirst, going to med school, and becoming a doctor. Med school was rigorous, fun, and delightful. It was also a total shit show, being the single fat young doctor in training.
>
> I always felt very exposed. At the end of my surgery clerkship, the clerkship director (a surgeon) told me I had done a good job and that the one thing I needed to do was get bariatric surgery quickly before I applied for residency. I had never

asked him to weigh in on any part of my health or my body. I had not solicited any feedback beyond what was demanded of me as a medical student training with him. He decided that I needed to lose weight. And to do it surgically. All I could come up with at the moment was that I couldn't afford it. And then he told me he would pay for it.

When we dehumanize fat bodies and call them wrong, disgusting, lazy, disease-prone, etc., not only are we inaccurate, we are also harming people, especially those who are fat. Fat people are devalued, stigmatized, disenfranchised, and victimized by prejudice and discrimination. They have diminished access to employment, raises, non-stigmatizing medical care, and basic respect. They can't go to a grocery store without dirty looks and food policing. Seats in restaurants, classrooms, public transportation, and airplanes do not accommodate all bodies. Fat people struggle to find affordable clothing to wear. Adolescents report weight as the most common reason for being bullied. And research shows all this impacts a fat person's health and well-being: experiencing pervasive weight stigma may actually be the cause of conditions we blame on high body weight: high blood pressure, insulin resistance, diabetes, abnormal cholesterol levels, and more. If we say we care about fat people's health, we should be paying attention to this.

Fat bodies are exploited by the diet, health, wellness, and fitness industries, and the academic, research, and health care communities collude with all of it. So it's no wonder that we are where we are today: 70 million people suffering with eating disorders worldwide, a $72 billion diet industry[4] with no data to support it, toxic "wellness" culture, and TV shows like *The Biggest Loser* and *1000-lb Sisters* that just reinforce stereotypes. We have a medical system with an enormous crisis of imagination when it comes to supporting the health and well-being of fat people. And researchers and academics, who've devoted their entire careers to a failed paradigm, remain unwilling to reckon with the data.

We said it in the Introduction and we will say it again: There is no evidence-based treatment for high body weight that leads to sustained weight loss five to ten years after the initial weight loss—and this includes weight loss surgeries.[5,6,7] The most consistent effect of weight loss after two years is weight gain. In fact, what we know from the failed weight loss paradigm is the best way to get people to gain weight over the course of their lifetime is by encouraging them to suppress their natural weight.

The truth is, bodies exist on a spectrum and come in a variety of presentations, abilities, shapes, and sizes. There have always been fat bodies and there always will be fat bodies, just as there have always been short bodies and tall bodies. Bodies are not supposed to fit into the narrow range stated in the BMI chart, and they are not meant to stay the same as we age. We should not be expected to weigh in our seventies what we weighed in our twenties. Bodies—and health—are always in flux, from the moment we are conceived in the womb until the moment we die. And we have far less control of both our health and our weight than we've been led to believe. Our focus needs a shift in direction. As Marilyn Wann has said, "The only thing that anyone can diagnose, with any certainty, by looking at a fat person, is their own level of stereotype and prejudice toward fat people."[8]

Now, at this point, you are probably sorting through all the things you believe you know about fatness, health, nutrition, etc., and looking for ways to reject our ideas. We are fairly certain that within an hour of setting this book down, you will receive messages that contradict and challenge what you are learning here and reinforce all the old messaging. So in this period of deep reckoning, you will likely find yourself straddling for a bit, with one foot over here in Body Trust and the other in the more familiar territory of Weight Watchers, Overeaters Anonymous (OA), etc. We get it. We know. We ask that you hang out here for a bit and see what you think as you learn more.

So why might you straddle? Because you believe you can't be trusted with food. And to that we want to say: Of course you don't trust yourself, given what you've been through, all that you've tried, and the way the diet, weight loss, cosmetic fitness, and wellness industries market their products and programs. If you've attended 12-step programs like OA or Food Addicts Anonymous, you've literally been told you can't be trusted. And the natural reaction to believing we can't be trusted is to pull the reins tighter by creating more restrictions, more rules, and more rigidity. In our desperation for some semblance of control, we look to outside experts to tell us what, when, and how much to eat. But over time, our tolerance to the *restrictions, rules, and rigidity* diminishes, and instead of thinking it is a sign of health that your body will not let you starve, you (and perhaps the people around you) believe there is something wrong with you and you just haven't found the right plan or tried hard enough. So it's back to the hustle, and the endless cycle of shame, self-blame, and striving for perfection persists.

Regardless of what has led you to this place of not trusting yourself, we want you to take a moment to pause and notice what initially drew you to this book. What have you read in these early pages that resonated for you? If you are like us and you like to highlight lines, mark up books, and make notes, what stood out to you? What has piqued your curiosity? Where have you heard truth?

Hold on to the pieces that are calling you and let that be enough right now. Something drew you to this book. Keep reading. And remember you can do what you want with the information in this book once you are done with it.

This work is countercultural and you will be misunderstood. If you share what you are learning here with people who have not done the work to understand how dominant culture has impacted them, they will think you are drinking the Kool-Aid! You might have to trust us on this one right now—*They are drinking the Kool-Aid*. So protect your process while you explore this work and deepen your own roots into body trust. You are learning a new language, and people who do not speak this language will not understand it, will tell you "it won't work," and will gaslight you.

As we've explored in this chapter a bit, you were born with a connection to and an inherent trust in your body. But the atmosphere in which we live and breathe is fueled by what founder of The Body Is Not an Apology and author of the book by the same name, Sonya Renee Taylor, calls "body terrorism." Along the way, you were socialized and habituated to leave your body and move through the world like a floating head. Body trust is disrupted by many things, including but not limited to trauma, oppression, illness, and social constructs of gender, race, sexuality, beauty, health, and weight. In an email to her newsletter subscribers, yoga teacher, author, and race-equity trainer Michelle C. Johnson writes:

> *Dominant culture doesn't want us to be in our bodies, let alone tune into our inner wisdom and knowing. Dominant culture wants us to move from our minds and thoughts, which the toxic culture has so deeply conditioned. When we operate from our neck up instead of our heart down, we move differently. My brain always tells me to speed up, and my heart says slow down, close your eyes and check in with yourself, and then respond.*

This book is an invitation to return to a relationship with your body and yourself that you want to be in for your lifetime—flexible, compassionate, and connected. As you divest from diet culture and root more deeply into body trust, you will:

* Experience more joy, freedom, ease, and satisfaction

* Increase the connection to your truth and your own knowing

* Have more strategies to navigate bad (body) days*

* Lean into foundational practices that don't require you to abandon yourself

---

* "Bad body days" are those days when you feel bad about your body or feel a strong pull to make a plan to restrict food.

* Feel more at home in your body

* Free up precious time and energy for more meaningful passions

We continue with Angela Braxton-Johnson's story:

> *Though my first few years of learning and practicing Body Trust wasn't easy, it was a necessary and restorative part of my journey, which continues today.*
>
> *I learned so many life-changing principles/theories. How diet culture was rooted in White Supremacy. About intersectionality. How to tap into my body's feelings and desires. How to be more compassionate with myself. How to aim for a C- rather than an A in how I live. About the ridiculousness of weight stigma. How my issues were not my fault. I also learned how to cuss a little bit. How to live for Angela (not everyone else) and let those delicious chips fall where they may.*
>
> *Most importantly, I've learned to embrace ALL of me! My Blackness. My Womanness. My Fatness. My Spirituality. My Creativity. My Everything. However my body decides to be! All while honoring this sacred temple in a way that's organically nourishing for me.*

Sounds pretty good, doesn't it?

Sometimes we begin with the awareness that we can't keep doing what we've been doing. Even when you want to keep hustling, your body may be done. Especially if it has become next to impossible to pull off the food plans for more than a few days or a few weeks. (Remember, this is a sign of health!) So begin by acknowledging that you can't go back, even though you don't know how to go forward. Reading this book will introduce you to new possibilities, and our hope is that it will help you move forward.

CHAPTER 2

Your Body Story

I hope you will go out and let stories happen to you,
and that you will work them, water them with your
blood and tears and your laughter till they bloom,
till you yourself burst into bloom.

—CLARISSA PINKOLA ESTÉS

We wonder what your mind conjures when you hear the term "body story." Maybe you imagine the kind of assignment you might get from a therapist but never actually do. Or perhaps you picture a bunch of privileged white women at an expensive retreat somewhere, talking about everything but the hardest thing. Or maybe it sounds like something people who have really suffered might think about, not at all like you.

Body stories, our real ones, are essentially missing. We are often reluctant to dive into our body stories because we believe they are too taboo to share or too boring to be of interest or value. Either way, our stories can become buried within us, layered beneath the stories we are indoctrinated into. Our body stories are not even wholly evident to us, instead covered up by ideas, efforts, and beliefs about how to constantly self-improve or acquiesce to mainstream ideas of health and beauty.

We are always surprised to notice that when new people join us at a Body Trust workshop or retreat, they are genuinely relieved to find that other group members have also been in a collective silence about how they are hustling in response to body shame. Our lack of stories has kept us from each other.

Aubrey Gordon, author of *What We Don't Talk About When We Talk About Fat*, says "When we reduce fat people to their bodies, to 'before and after,' or to bellies and rolls, we come to think of fat people as bodies without personhood. Fat bodies become symbols of disembodied disgust."[1]

When have you read the story of living in a fat body that was not told through a diet program or a TV show like *1000-lb Sisters* or *The Biggest Loser*? What about the true story of living in a fat body? Have you ever? Where are the stories of fatness? They are subjugated and pushed underground.

We need more stories from those who have defied the standard narrative of body apology and demand care, dignity, and respect. What of the bodies who live their lives with illness or disability or chronic pain? Or what of sharing validating stories of what it means to claim one's struggle with disordered eating in a nonbinary or trans body when the construct of gender is the true trauma? What if we heard more stories like those from James Baldwin, Ta-Nehisi Coates, and Toni Morrison that speak to a culture that denies the impacts of racism, weight stigma/fatphobia, ableism, transphobia, etc., and thus the lived experience of moving through the world without a sense of safety because of marginalized identities? What would we learn if we heard these stories? What if these stories were not relegated to therapists' offices and other such private conversations? We need the stories to get us all closer to our own as well as others' humanity and further from The Hustle. These stories have the power to change how we regard all bodies.

We need to hear more body stories to be less alone in our own. Alone can be where ideas of good and bad, worthy or not worthy, give rise to disordered relationships with food and the body. This is where diet culture counts on capitalizing and recycling itself, trusting you to blame yourself instead of The Plan (food, exercise, etc.). In the loneliness, our efforts at coping and surviving can lead to feeling increasingly fragmented, and it is when we feel fragmented, facilitator and consultant Desiree Adaway says, that we are easier to control. Control is often a compelling path in our struggles with our bodies. Control can feel like the answer to the deep inner separation that comes from cycling through bouts with dieting and disordered eating again and again. Control seemingly offers clarity, a path forward, and a plan. And no matter how you slice it, control is an illusion. We are here for more than stories of what we controlled, restrained, pulled off, and performed. We need real human body stories to heal and move forward.

As we mentioned, we've watched with utter amazement as folks who gather with us in retreats and groups begin to understand, for the very first time, that others are having an experience similar to theirs. Others are also bingeing, hiding food and eating in secret, purging, or compulsively exercising. They believe anything they eat is too much. That they are fucked up about all of it. No one is confidently "getting it right" for more than a few months at a time and they don't know why. The truth is, you may be less alone than you think.

Here's how one common weight control story goes. We think we want change for a while, and then something pushes us toward trying something new. So we grab on to an eating plan we've heard about, or a "lifestyle change." We get a lift, we feel better. That sense of "control" reenters. It's a relief. It's measurable—we know whether or not we are "doing it right." We lean into our most stringent, perfectionistic self to hold us accountable to the plan. We go along. We think any ambivalence we feel about it is a sign of weakness. We work to hold the weakness at bay. Life happens, as it inevitably does, and we lose the thread of the plan and feel like shit about ourselves again. This shitty feeling is the one that grasping for control was distancing us from in the beginning. The sense of weakness or shame about ourselves and our inability to conquer the frustrations with food and our body is who we are afraid we truly are.

Remember, restrictive eating plans were never going to work. It's not you. Our bodies have strong physiological and psychological responses to food deprivation (more on this later). They just aren't great at it over the long term. These plans often need disdain and self-loathing. They rely on your surviving and striving self, instead of your rooted or thriving self. They call on the parts of you that want to seal up the internal and scary broken bits with something that looks smooth and shiny on the outside but leaves the inside raw and untended.

Having the perfect body is a pursuit we are introduced to in formative years. We learn, often before puberty, that the body can be changed, and should be changed if there is the presence of fat. We see these ideas in our family and friends, on buses and social media ads. We hear more about weight loss than we do about eating disorders, despite their commonality *and* lethality. In response to what we commonly are taught about eating disorders, we believe "too skinny" is the primary problem—not the starvation or malnutrition or compulsive exercise or the physical and psychological harm that occurs in people of all sizes who have eating disorders.

All roads lead to this: We believe the body is akin to a formative putty if we follow the rules. We learn weight loss is a good thing, and pulling it off is a triumph and is also required to be respected. This is where we are likely to integrate the value of restriction and restraint over eating to meet our needs. When it comes to stories of fatness and the body, we are hard pressed to find stories that do not contain the seductive narrative arc of weight loss, as if this is enough to make a body, thus a human existence, redeem itself. Our needs are suspect in this narrative. Our bodies are controllable, but only if we master control over ourselves.

Control is the lie. It is the promise that comes through whiteness and dominant culture; it appeases the patriarchy; it is fodder for those who sell solutions to the problem of fatness without ever acknowledging the aftermath of pain that leads to internal fragmentation, weight regain, and body blame. It holds the exterior part of us together on the outside, leaving no clues to the struggle on the inside. We can try to go about our lives as cogs in the system, as capitalism intends, because if you are making it work on the outside, fewer people will encounter the feelings of chaos, disorder, or shame that dominate your inner world. We get further disconnected from our truth. Our stories are told from the outside in, instead of the inside out.

Understanding the experiences, stories, and circumstances that contributed to how you lost trust with your body is an important element of healing. Shelby Gordon, a Body Trust Coach and equity consultant, shared what working with her body story has meant to her. She said,

> *Exploring my body story is my healing, because it gives me permission to look at all of these nooks and crevices, all of these Mount Everest–like mountains and all of the pebbles in my own time, in my own way, at my own pace, and at my own depth. My body story involves generational trauma, ancestral trauma. It involves purity culture. It involves narcissism. It involves single child syndrome. It involves burlesque and sensuality and reengaging human functions that I had denied. That I just cut out of my life. And it's given me permission to explore how that happened, why it happened, and set a path to heal.*

Remember, our bodies have been with us through everything we've experienced in our lives. They hold the stories and experiences of our people. They are a constant presence, companion, and witness to life. With us for every breath we've taken . . . every beat of our heart. Our body has survived our scrutiny, our shame. It has been impacted by the oppressive ideas fed to us about what our bodies symbolize to others. There is so much more to say.

In the previous chapter, we offered some questions to help you begin to explore your body story. A foundational question we want you to consider right now is:

When did I learn my body was a problem? How old was I, where was I, and who was I with?

Our body shame has roots. Some of the body stories we share in this book highlight when the first seeds were planted. Rachael, who is mixed race, was asked by random adults throughout her childhood, "What are you?" and while she didn't know exactly what this meant, she remembers feeling threatened by the question. Aaron recalls the day he realized his body was different while playing sports, validating his belief that his body was never going to be "elite" or good enough to be an athlete. Anna was in the dressing room with her mother when she saw the pain and disappointment on her mother's face when they couldn't find clothes to fit her ten-year-old body.

One of the core phases of reclaiming body trust is to explore your body story to understand the experiences in your life that have disrupted your sense of belonging or trust with your body—and where shame took root. Understanding how we lose trust in our bodies helps us locate the problem outside of our bodies, clearing the way for new personal narratives to emerge. We deserve agency over the telling of our truth. We are the only ones who can truly write our story. Author Lidia Yuknavitch writes:

I am not the story you made of me. You are not the story they made of you. We are not the story they made of us. Take the stories back. Restory.[2]

Body stories, *our* stories, cannot be predetermined or even predicted, though you have likely encountered many people who have tried. Body stories are not meant to be prescriptions, either: only believed and understood if redemptive. Our stories desire to exist as both simultaneously complex and mundane as they can be. Not calculated by size, race, ethnicity, citizenship status, gender, age, sexuality, religion, health status, or ability. Our stories, the truth of our own lived experience, want to be heard, witnessed, and held as evidence of a life lived against the odds in a world that does not love or trust all bodies. We want to exist in possibility, not limited by dominant ideals of how much space we get to take up or how we are allowed to exist in this world.

If you think of the stories you do hear, the story lines may feel like tropes. Like the stories of trauma being healed through bootstrapping and perseverance. Or problematized, scapegoated bodies that ultimately are accepted and made peace with. Maybe you've heard stories where the person who had a fat body ends up thinner or "healthier"—a redemptive, "happy" ending. Or the stories that show people working hard to "better" themselves through "health," rescuing themselves from the negative outcomes of their so-called transgressions. This is an overemphasis on false goodness.

On the rare occasion we do see fat people on screen, the characters they play have historically had weight as a central issue, which only reinforces shame and anti-fat bias. Some of you may remember Fat Monica on *Friends*, an exaggerated caricature of a fat person, often seen stuffing her face with food and making a mess while eating. There was an episode where she danced with a donut. And her brother Ross fat-shamed her throughout the series with comments about her past body. One episode imagined what life would have been like for her had she never lost weight, with the primary story line being that she'd still be a virgin.

Chrissy Metz, the fat actress on the acclaimed TV show *This Is Us*, has spoken publicly about how weight loss was an expectation when she signed on to play Kate. While there weren't specific numbers or a time frame, she and the show's creator have shared that they discuss the plan for Kate as well as Metz's own goals about once every year.[3] Then you have Rebel Wilson's character, Fat Amy, in *Pitch Perfect*, who plays the stereotypically fat sidekick. And the characters on the TV series *Mike & Molly* met at Overeaters Anonymous, because clearly this is the only place two fat people would meet and fall in love.

Can we collectively consider why a fat person needs to be portrayed as obsessed with their weight when it is actually the world around the fat body that is obsessed, narrating and then profiting off the narrations? Stories from fat people who are living their lives despite diet culture and anti-fat bias are just an internet search away. The upholders of these narratives don't trust us to evolve past our body shame. And the harm this causes is virtually invisible to the mainstream world. But it is the main event in our private practices.

In more recent years, we've had some improvement in the portrayal of fat people, and even story lines that challenge the cultural narrative of what it means to be fat. *Booksmart*'s Beanie Feldstein's character, Molly, who is average in size but considered fat by movie standards, never talks about her weight, nor was she shamed for her size in any scene (very different from what we are used to seeing). The TV show *Shrill*, based on the book by Lindy West, follows Aidy Bryant's character as she reckons with the harm incurred by living in a culture steeped in anti-fat bias, a mother who focused on her weight growing up, and the realization that she doesn't have to lose weight to live a happy, fulfilling life. How radical! We recently watched the Netflix movie *Thunder Force* with Melissa McCarthy and Octavia Spencer, two actors who've spoken up in the past about the challenges they have faced finding designers to dress them for the red carpet. They play two fat superheroes whose weight isn't brought up as a barrier even once in the story line. How might our body stories be different if more narratives like these existed in pop culture?

We are not often told our bodies are trustworthy. We believe trusting our bodies may ultimately get us into trouble. Some act as if bodies are essentially childlike, and they take on a self-parenting style most of us would reject for any child. We act as if our bodies need discipline, some tough love and firm star charts to keep them from perpetually acting out. If we are inconsistent in our approach, our bodies may falter and we will feel shame or apology for letting ourselves go. If we don't follow through, we are making excuses, and if we don't change despite our efforts, we need to try harder.

This approach mirrors the way the dominant culture considers trauma, hardship, and suffering, which is to say it doesn't. The trauma of living in a Black, brown, fat, nonbinary or trans, sick, disabled, or female body is not enough to challenge the cultural construct, the cultural story of rising above, persevering, and being successful in regard to the body. Redeeming ourselves and *shining* is the story we are used to. The rest? Disregarded, disbelieved, and brushed under the rug.

As children, we inherit our stories—and more specifically, the framing of them. The fairy tales and even archetypes we are exposed to may teach us about possibilities for our lives but do not necessarily reveal what it is like to actually live our lives in our body. In truth, our efforts are messy as can be, rarely follow a linear path, do not exist well in a binary, and we tend to think it is over if we arrive at our idealized destination. Probably because the path felt more like jumping through hoops or trying to please or was simply exhausting. Maybe because we did not become more of ourselves, but likely more of what we thought was expected of us to experience worthiness or belonging. When we hustle for health in this culture, is it a hustle for a sense of well-being? Or is it a hustle for worthiness? More so, isn't this hustle for belonging, for acceptance, and for being understood as real and vital?

How has your body, just as it is, helped you survive in the world?

You've survived living in a culture that encouraged you to act violently upon your body in order to fit into narrowly defined standards of beauty and worth. We are speaking about starvation, self-hate, visions of self-mutilation, denial of pleasure and desire, turning some bodies asexual because they don't meet cultural ideals of desirability, negative energy balances, trading your voice and presence to avoid weight stigma, and on and on. Often prescribed and endorsed by the culture, medicine, and loved ones, this is violence and aggression against a human body, pure and simple. These acts are sometimes the wisest coping mechanisms available in a culture that distrusts you and hates your body. They can be as self-preserving as they are aggressive. They are sometimes exactly what we have to do to get through uncertain, challenging, and traumatizing times. These forms of coping also numb us, keep us in compliance, reinforce internalized self-blame for something that was never ours, turn growing rage in on ourselves because the culture will not metabolize it, and help us try to keep our bodies in check so we will be loved, hired, respected, and included. We have all contributed to this dilemma in one way or another. And we all are responsible for correcting this harm.

If you see yourself in this, let us ask . . . is the above story congruent with the one you tell yourself? What would a story told through a lens of truth, self-respect, or self-love sound like? How would it differ? Whose telling of your body story can you trust?

Your body has underscored your very perception of what it means to be you . . . and to be alive. Your body holds your emotions, your loves and losses, your fears and struggles, your desires, your creative juices, your ideas, your hopes, your expression of DNA and intergenerational trauma. It holds you. You are your body. Your body has its own story—a story of resistance and resilience—told through memories, sensations, emotions, and intuition. It's a story of survival, and it deserves to be told, heard, and witnessed. By you and for you.

We live for the day when we are rapt with attention for understanding how the stories—your stories in fact, that have not been heard and understood—will be centered, and the telling of stories that sell body improvement disguised with health claims will be publicly deemed as hollow as we may feel when we try to relate to them.

What do you wish the world knew about your body?

How did you survive and become you?

What is the story of your body surviving in this world?

We re-story as an act of reclamation. We grab our stories from the clutches of what is supposed to be and infuse them with the truth—all the pieces dominant culture has hidden from view, has explained away for you, or has made invisible.

The re-storying of our experience helps us gain awareness of what was our coping, our protection, our efforts to survive and to make our way. We begin to see what belongs to us and what never did. You keep what you want, or maybe you whittle away at the lies over time. What once may have been considered failure may be forgiven. What once was a feeling of never enough may become a conduit of reconnection to all that you have been and done to make your life meaningful, purposeful, and enough. Ultimately, we want you left with your bare truth, un-apologetic, with shame loosened and left to the wayside, and agency and power reclaimed without seeking permission to do so.

Claim it all. And begin to tell the truest story.

BODY TRUST AND TRANS EXPERIENCE

by Sand Chang

Dearest Trans and/or Nonbinary Siblings, Sisters, Brothers,

I offer this letter to you. When I say "you," I mean anyone who is trans, and/or nonbinary, or for whom cisnormative culture and expectations simply do not apply but are applied anyway. I am writing to you even if you don't have the words for how to describe your gender all the time (I sure don't). I am writing to you if you have a strong connection to being trans, if you ever feel like you're not trans enough, if binary conceptions of gender fail to honor the truth of who you are, if you think colonialist conceptions of transgender experience are bullshit, or all of the above.

You may be wondering if all this talk of body trust applies to you. You may be accustomed to having to do the mental gymnastics of stretching what is typically written by and for cis people to determine what fits for you and how it relates to your trans body. You may be thinking that Body Trust is for cis people, for white people, for anyone who has a chance of having a "good" body if they only lost weight.

I don't have all the answers, and I won't presume to understand your exact experience. Isn't that part of the problem? Trying to force understanding through a universal trans narrative so that everyone else doesn't have to learn how to listen or expand their ideas about gender? What I can offer is one perspective based on the intersections of lived experience and being professionalized in that experience. On one hand, I am a queer, nonbinary, Chinese American with a long history of severe restriction, compulsive exercise, orthorexia, and body shame/shaming. On the other hand, I am a licensed mental health provider whose degrees, certifications, and accomplishments gain me access to being recognized in largely white, cis, gatekeeping systems. And as a person who acknowledges the multiplicity of being many things at once, sometimes in ways that are seemingly contradictory, both of these aspects of my experience give me insight while neither makes me an expert.

What can I say to you about gender and Body Trust that you don't already know?

I can give you facts and figures and research citations. I can tell you that even though there is a myth that eating disorders affect only white cis heterosexual women, trans people are actually over eight times more likely than cis women to have been diagnosed with an eating disorder.[1] This is likely an underestimate given that the measurement (including diagnosis) of eating disorders is so stringent and culturally biased that most of us who suffer from them will never meet full criteria for a diagnosis. Part of me wants to say fuck diagnosis, but I also know that having a diagnosis is often the ticket to accessing health care services. I can tell you that X amount of Y kinds of trans people report a certain assortment of behaviors, thoughts, feelings, and sensations Z percent of the time and that virtually no one knows what the fuck to do about it. Sometimes "data" is validating, while at others it is alienating and exclusionary.

And then there's the question of whether the concept of having an eating disorder even applies when it is our world itself that is disordered with white supremacy, anti-Blackness, colonialism, transphobia, fatphobia, ableism, and the list goes on. It's hard to have a body. It's even harder to have a body that is perpetually under appraisal, surveillance, or attack. Even though we have agency, ultimately we do not have control over how others perceive or treat us, even the most well-meaning of friends, family members, coworkers, or strangers. Sometimes these pressures come from other trans and nonbinary people; it's what happens when trauma responds by tearing others down when we need to be holding collective space to heal for each other. It makes sense, then, given all of these factors, that many of us turn to certain behaviors to survive, cope, numb out, or create an illusion of control to manage our physical and emotional pain.

I don't actually believe that disordered eating shows up in trans bodies the same way that it does for cis bodies. It may look similar on the outside in terms of *behaviors* such as food restriction, binge eating, compulsive exercise, or purging. But what's on the *inside* is different. It's rarely about wanting our bodies to look a certain way just for aesthetics or desirability. It's about safety. It's about wanting to feel seen as human beings. It's about ways that we find a sense of control when we don't have access to the things that will help us to feel well, secure. It's about lack of accessibility to food, whether early in life or in our current lives, that sets us up to have a complicated, unpredictable relationship with food. It's about coping with anti-trans bias, discrimination, rejection, isolation. It's about survival.

I invite you to trust your own lived experience. Despite our medical and mental health systems doing everything they can to control our narratives, to tell us who we are, or to judge whether we are enough of who we are, we are the holders of truth in our lives. Despite colonialism and white supremacy telling us that there is a right way to have a gender, our lived experience tells us otherwise. It tells the truth. If you have struggled with eating or the shape or size of your body, then no diagnostic manual or person with letters after their name can tell you whether you deserve to receive care or tend to the parts of you that are hurting.

Easier said than done, you might say. Bear with me.

When I learned about Body Trust, I didn't realize that it wasn't just about food or my weight or diet culture. Body Trust goes beyond intuitive eating or monitoring our hunger and fullness cues.

It is about a deep listening to our selves. And when we truly start to listen, we cannot be selective.

When I started to listen to my body and feelings about gender, the ones that finally spoke to me the things I already knew in my heart of hearts, I could not drown out the other truths that emerged. And when I truly let myself feel the grief and rage that resulted from the trauma of receiving health care that was indifferent to my needs as a nonbinary person, I started to open up to healing from my eating disorder. It hasn't been cute or graceful in any way. In fact, it's been messy and confusing as hell. Some of the confusion I felt actually stemmed from anti-diet or body positive movements. I didn't know how to make sense of the "just accept yourself" or "love your body" statements (mostly from white cis het thin women!). These sentiments didn't land easily on this body of mine that I had been taught to hate. Was that hatred a sin? When did compulsory self-love become the new morality?

I'm not going to tell you to look in the mirror and say, "I love you." Not if the words don't mean anything. Not if it's a form of bypassing the parts of us that need to hear that it's okay to not be okay. To not feel okay. To not love or even like ourselves every day. To feel so many complicated feelings about our bodies that are sometimes about gender and sometimes not.

I'm also not going to tell you that you need to challenge your "distorted" thoughts or find the "evidence" against your feelings so that you gaslight yourself. That, to me, is the opposite of body trust. In diet culture, the mind is a tool for subjugating the body, telling it when and how to eat and move and rest regardless of what the body actually needs. It's all about mind over matter. This doesn't work, not for food and exercise and relating to our weight or size, and it sure as hell does not work for gender. We cannot will ourselves to feel differently about our gender, or be cisgender like people want us to be, or shut off our experiences of dysphoria. So many of us have tried to do just this, which in the end has prolonged and increased dysphoria, suffering, depression, anxiety, and more.

What I will encourage you to do is to get honest with yourself about what is and isn't working for you. I know it's complicated. Sometimes there are things that work in the moment that don't end up working out for us longer term. You might think that what you are doing is reducing dysphoria, and maybe it does—until it doesn't. Sometimes the things that are helping us to survive emotional pain actually cause harm to our bodies or our health. If you are in fact engaging in disordered eating, whether it be restriction or binge eating or purging or compulsive exercise or something else, I encourage you to think about it from the lens of harm reduction and to consider what it is you really need. Here are some questions to ask yourself: *What are the benefits of doing what I'm doing? What are the costs? What are the deeper needs that I am trying to get met? Is there someone I can go to for support, even if it's just telling them that I am struggling? Are there things that I cannot change that I need help coping with or accepting? Are there things that need to change but cannot because of external constraints or my own inner blocks? What is appropriate for me at this time?*

I also encourage you to look for the moments, however brief, when you feel neutral to positive feelings about your body. Maybe there are moments of gender euphoria or gendergood that you are able to access. Not in some toxic positivity way, not as a way to deny the fact that dysphoria or body discomfort exist. In somatic therapy approaches, there is a concept called "pendulation" that is the process by which we shift between states of arousal and states of calm in order to find balance or regulation. Finding these moments or touchpoints where we can connect to an inner or external resource can make all the difference. For me that's being with my dogs, taking pictures of my dogs, dressing my dogs up in clothes, well . . . you get the point. *Where do you find glimpses of joy? Can you give yourself permission to feel into that joy even if you're in pain?*

Other things I cannot emphasize enough for those of you who are seeking formal or professional eating disorders treatment:

1. You may never fit the mold of eating disorders recovery that is presented to or expected of you, so FUCK THAT. Your recovery has to look and feel the way it needs to for you, not for anyone else who expects you to follow some cookie cutter treatment plan that was designed for someone else.

2. It is not your job to educate your medical and mental health providers about gender or trans people. Your providers are getting *paid* to do their job, and they need to take responsibility for gaining the knowledge, awareness, and skills necessary to serve you or anyone else who shows up as a client.

3. You do not have to center cis people's comfort over your own.

4. Getting better *does* require you to take certain actions or change certain behaviors on your own behalf (essentially, to find ways to engage meaningfully with your own recovery process), but individual behaviors or choices will never be the full picture when it comes to health, healing, or recovery. Systems need to change to support you. When I say systems, I'm talking about everything from a treatment center's capacity to provide affirming care, to gatekeeping medical systems, to larger systems of oppression: anti-trans bias, anti-fat bias, ableism, white supremacy, capitalism, colonialism, and classism, to name a few.

5. Find community. There are more and more people talking about their lived experiences being trans and/or nonbinary and struggling with food or their bodies. Remember that you

are not alone. And that recovery is easier if you are able to find people whose experiences are closer to or even mirror yours.

As a community we are still finding each other and ourselves. I hope that reading this letter has helped you even a little. It takes time to build trust in our bodies, and maybe having 100 percent trust isn't the goal. It's not a destination or a place to arrive at for once and for good. If a sense of trust, if only what feels like one percent of a feeling of trust, can be found in a fleeting moment, sometimes that can be enough to help us get by. Again, it might be messy, painful, confusing. Even then, I wish for you to find some comfort in these words:

You are enough. You belong.
You are enough. You belong.
You are enough. You belong.

In love and struggle,

Sand Chang

Sand Chang, PhD (they/them/their), is a Chinese American, genderfluid, nonbinary psychologist and trauma-informed DEI consultant residing on unceded Ohlone land also known as Oakland, California. They are a Certified Body Trust Provider, Certified IFS therapist, and Certified EMDR therapist. Their career has been dedicated to body liberation, specifically with regards to trans health, eating disorders, and trauma. They coauthored *A Clinician's Guide to Gender-Affirming Care: Working with Transgender and Gender Nonconforming Clients* (New Harbinger, 2018). Outside of work, Sand is a dancer, punoff competitor, and smoosh-faced-dog enthusiast.

Note: We have other letters on our website for readers of this book, including one for parents and caregivers, teachers and school administrators, and health care providers and helping professionals.

CHAPTER 3

Your Coping Is Rooted in Wisdom

*Transformation doesn't happen in a linear way,
at least not one we can always track. It happens in cycles,
convergences, explosions. If we release the framework
of failure, we can realize that we are in iterative cycles,
and we can keep asking ourselves—
how do I learn from this?*

—adrienne maree brown, *EMERGENT STRATEGY*

O ur body stories help us illustrate the bridge between how our lived experience has informed our coping. Body Trust participant Jen Inaldo shared some of her story with us:

I remember watching Tricia do a cartwheel during recess in third grade. I found a grassy spot and tried to do one and the results were not the same.

"You just do it like this!" She did another cartwheel. Hands up, arms straight, fling body to the side and throw legs over. "Just watch me. Just do it!"

I raised my hands over my head. I looked to my side and I tried to will my legs up and over, but the moment my hands touched the ground, my legs decided they did not want to cartwheel and I crumbled to the ground. I remember sitting there for a moment to get my bearings, to see if anything hurt.

"That's okay," Tricia said, standing over me. "My mom's fat too, and she can't do cartwheels, either."

Wait. What?

This is my earliest memory of having a body.

It was surprisingly easy for me to stuff this memory away. It was also surprisingly easy to say, "I'm not hungry anymore," when I was definitely hungry but I didn't want to finish a meal. I don't know if I ever put two and two together. A set of rules I had not even been aware of entered my life and revealed themselves in these tiny actions. Don't clean your plate unless they make you. Don't ask for seconds. Some foods were good and some were bad and if you wanted the bad stuff you have to eat that in the bathroom or at night when everyone is asleep, where no one can see you. If you can get away with it, don't tuck your shirt in because then people can see the shape of your belly and how it poofs out.

Our culture does not expect us to occupy the bodies we actually have and upholds a constant stream of options for fixing fixing fixing. In the context of diet culture, we are handed a seemingly simple solution: control your hungers, desires, body. In essence, participation in diet culture becomes our coping. Acquiescing becomes our coping. Doing things *to and on* our bodies instead of *for and with* feels more possible than resisting objectification. Living in a culture that places bodies in a hierarchy that impacts our sense of ourselves and how we engage with the world requires us to find ways to cope. The ways we learn to cope have been rooted in wisdom: the wisdom that teaches us how to survive body-based oppression. These coping patterns—the ways you have learned to push past your basic needs (hunger, fatigue, connection, desire) to change your body, keep up, maintain control, or chase worthiness—help you keep going. The harm these methods cause gets buried beneath our individual efforts at a solution and the cultural narrative that these efforts are good for you. When you take a closer look, these practices are really about whose bodies are valued.

In *You Are Your Best Thing*, an anthology of Black experience edited by Tarana Burke and Brené Brown, Burke says, in the introduction to the book,

> *We often carry our trauma in similar ways, but the roads that led us to the trauma are all so different. We must pay attention to that road. That road is our humanity. That road is the piece that we are talking about. A lot of times, we're happy and relieved to find similarities: "Oh, you too? You too? Me too." No pun intended. These experiences create community, and it's wonderful, but it is still critical to understand the very different paths that led you to the trauma.*

In the previous chapter, we talked about how we rarely hear stories that diverge from the main road. In the world of healing, "wellness," and eating disorder treatment, this translates into having few to no programs and services that people of color, fat folks, trans and nonbinary and disabled folks can see themselves in. Jen's words illustrate this difference:

> *The world is not safe for fat bodies.*
>
> *Not only am I fat, I am also not white. I am very self-aware. Even though I am socially awkward, I can read the room very well. I'm always second-guessing what I'm wearing. I've only once been able to fit into a pair of pants from Express. This was a thing. This used to be a measurement. There was a point in my life I could wear the largest size at Express, but the mate-*

rial hugged me and emphasized where my belly separates into two distinct hemispheres. Even at my smallest, my belly has always been cut into two, one donut sitting on top of another.

I had always thought that if I was five inches taller this would all even itself out and my life would be different.

This is not true. I know it's ridiculous to think this, but I can't help but wonder how much easier it would be, outside of just being able to reach things off higher shelves.

All my problems fixed forever with just five more inches of height.

The mythical taller thin me is never going to exist. Not in this lifetime or another.

When I was in my late teens I made her up. I saw her for the very first time in a dELiA's catalogue. She was slightly taller than I was (five inches! It's just five inches!). She was rocking some awesome pigtails and a pair of joggers and a crop top. She had black hair and white skin with only a tiny inkling of eye makeup. She looked confident and fun and likable.

I'm still reconciling that all idealized versions of me I could imagine were white. This is not a mistake considering my life was mostly John Hughes movies and prime time television. As far as pop culture was concerned, I did not exist. Fat. Southeast Asian. Short. Not particularly spunky enough to be a faithful sidekick. I could not connect to my body because I didn't want to live in it and the culture kept selling me the idea I could have the one I wanted if I just tried harder.

I'd like to think that things have gotten better. Some things have, but the fact that skin lightening creams are still being made means people are still buying them, which means people still want out of the bodies they currently have.

Sometimes I do too. On hard days I just want a smaller white body so people will leave me alone.

Trauma lives in our bodies. Everything we survive and endure happens in our bodies, whether we are able to be in them or not. When we talk about trauma, we don't just mean singular events of harm or violation. We also mean the institutional and systemic harm that impacts how safe and free people are as they move about in the world. And the harm that comes from our relationships, when love is given and withdrawn, feels conditional or is inconsistent because of the intergenerational patterns of harm that our family members hold within them. Our bodies hold the trauma, and together, our body, mind, and spirit devise ways for us to survive. In his memoir *Heavy*, Kiese Laymon writes, "I thought about the safety I found in eating too much, eating too late, eating to run away from memory. I stopped eating red meat, then pork, then chicken, then fish. I stopped eating eggs, then bread, then anything with refined sugar. I started running at night. I added three hundred push-ups a day. Then three hundred sit-ups . . . losing weight made me feel like I was from the future, like I could literally fly away from folk when I wanted to. Heavy was yesterday."

Your pattern or cycle of coping has been informed by all the ways you have creatively made your way in this world. The Cycle is made of actions, behaviors, and plans to address the inadequacies you perceive about your body, your food choices, your life. These negative beliefs have built themselves into the background of your life, driving, planning, enforcing, and putting limits on full access to yourself and your ability to own and embrace your value. The Cycle has likely impacted your sense of competency in your own care, as well as trust in your body and yourself. Uncovering your Cycle reveals how this wise coping has worked in subtle and not-so-subtle ways. We hope this chapter helps illuminate some parts of your pattern. With this increased awareness, you will begin to see new possibilities for transforming The Cycle and ways to rebuild trust with yourself again.

It wouldn't be unusual, though, if you are thinking, "I'm not exactly sure what they are talking about here. What coping? What patterns? I don't think I have any patterns." In her book, *The Politics of Trauma*, Staci K. Haines writes,

> *Recognizing our own survival strategies can, in and of itself, begin to open more choices. These behaviors may not be "who I am," but rather how I best adapted for safety, belonging, and dignity.*

This is how these patterns of coping operate. They often run just underneath our consciousness, keeping us protected, distracted, and surviving in a culture that demands we hustle and compete for our sense of worthiness. Sometimes we notice parts, we catch a glimpse of how our thoughts and feelings are driving our choices and reactions. We don't often see them in their entirety. And sometimes they aren't evident at all. It's all by design. The part most often visible is the part that exemplifies our striving—what we are doing to improve ourselves. The rest we may keep hidden or not consciously own. We want to separate ourselves from the parts we are most ashamed of, orphaning some of our coping as if it is an error or a misstep. But the thing about patterns is the various phases are in it together. It can't be fragmented. It works the way it does for a reason.

Body Trust participant Eva shared this about her process of understanding the ways food and body took center stage in her life, and talks about how elements of her mom's relationship with her own body took root in her body and patterns:

> *There were little nuanced ways my mom affected how I saw myself and really overt ways our relationship was destructive. A lot of subtle stuff was hard to get rid of, like how often she talked about her own body, how often she talked about trying to lose weight herself and then how much of that she put on me so young. I have memories going back to six, seven, eight years old. She would say things about my value and my worth as a physical person, especially from a sexuality standpoint.*

That women serve a purpose: to look good for men. I didn't realize how early that had started.

I've also realized how much she had taken away my own voice early on. A big part of repairing myself later came when I was able to stand up for myself. I remember doing things like telling my boss, "I just can't do this night shift anymore." Or my husband, "You gotta accept me the way I am. I'm not going to change for you anymore." I got to a point where I could just say no, that's not who I am. That's not what I'm going to do. It's not who I want to be. That's not the life I want to live. My mom taught me that the only acceptable behavior was people-pleasing all the time and that's intense.

The Cycle operates as a *predictable* pattern of thoughts, feelings, sensations, and behaviors that repeat over and over again, reinforcing shame, self-blame, and disordered eating behavior. It often begins with an eating behavior you call The Problem, which is followed by an onslaught of shame (The Shame Shitstorm) before you make The Plan to rescue you from yourself. The Plan creates some hope and distances you from shame before Life ultimately disrupts The Plan and sends you right back to The Problem. Understanding your cycle is a compassionate way to uncover your inner workings and see why it has been a struggle to trust yourself and your body. The Cycle is also a major clue into what your relationship with food has been doing for you.

Nicole K. continues with her body story:

At age twenty-three, I was a newly married, first-year teacher who had moved across the country so my husband could go to grad school. During this time, he joined a band and started touring, and this is when my full-fledged eating disorder began. I returned to the comfort of what I knew as a child, only this time it overtook my life. Bingeing became an everyday occurrence. I was so lonely and eating became my lifeline, my friend.

I began to gain weight. The more I hated how I looked, the more I ate to numb my feelings. The more I ate, the more weight I gained and the more I hated myself. I felt absolutely helpless.

⇢⋙ The Cycle ⋘⇠

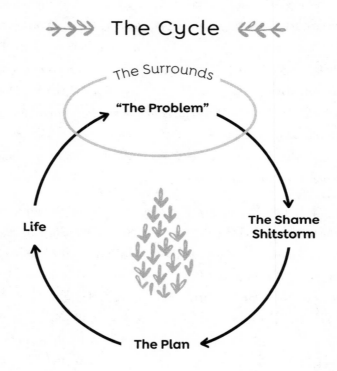

When people like Nicole seek support, they are often lured into restrictive food plans or a weight loss program that just adds fuel to The Cycle because the real problem (loneliness in Nicole's case) remains unaddressed. There may be some temporary relief and a belief that it can (and will) be different with this new plan. When The Plan changes as you evolve the ways in which you are trying to fix The Problem, it can be difficult to see that your cycle is repetitive. Remember, a big part of the pattern is blaming yourself for failing instead of understanding all the ways these plans were never really designed to work for you.

The pattern includes how you have treated yourself over time and what you believe about yourself deep down inside. If you fear or believe you have *less value unless you (or your body) change*, then you have likely been (understandably) acting out a pattern of thoughts, feelings, and behaviors that are all about making yourself better.

The lure of self-improvement—or treating yourself like a project or a problem to be solved—is the undercurrent of The Cycle and inserts itself into every part of your life. What if you did not need to fix yourself? What if this journey is about opening yourself to the wholeness that is alive and present in your body right now? Body Trust is a radical re-visioning of what it means to occupy and care for the body. If we believe we began as whole and have been distanced from our wholeness due to coping and survival, it is much easier to consider trusting the wisdom that comes from within. Who would you be if you weren't always planning the next step on your Body Project?

Shay's Body Story

Shay doesn't remember a time when she liked or felt at home in her body. Shay is a creative person who loves her job, her partner, her pets, and her friends. She recalls growing up in a family of people who were always working on losing weight or changing some aspect of their body. A gathering would always be full of apology for eating and plans for changing. People talked about other people's bodies and the way someone's body got bigger or smaller in knowing tones. They didn't talk about feelings or their relationships with each other as much as they talked about bodies. Everyone was fatphobic, but they said it was about health. And it felt bad for reasons that were hard to name. This felt nothing like health. Shay began to notice when her family complimented her and when they didn't. Her weight and her worthiness were increasingly fused. And she couldn't see her way out of it.

Shay grew up in a home where SlimFast cans and Diet Coke were regulars in the cabinet. Focusing on changing her body was often encouraged—she was invited for jogs and Weight Watchers meetings. It was a surefire way to connect with other women in her family.

Shay had "tried every diet ever put on the market." She'd lost weight, meeting her goal a couple of times, and the weight would always come back, plus more. Shay believed it was her fault she couldn't keep her weight down. She was frustrated and also finding that she could no longer stick to a plan for more than a few days. She felt like a failure and wondered if she was ever going to get this right. It was the one area of her life where she felt like she couldn't "pull it together."

When Shay started to think about her cycle, emotional eating and binge eating were the things she said were The Problem. These behaviors always messed with her ultimate goal. She felt like a "disgusting mess" whenever she thought she was eating off plan or "unhealthy," and she was always thinking of ways she needed to compensate. She was exhausted. Here's a more detailed picture of Shay's cycle:

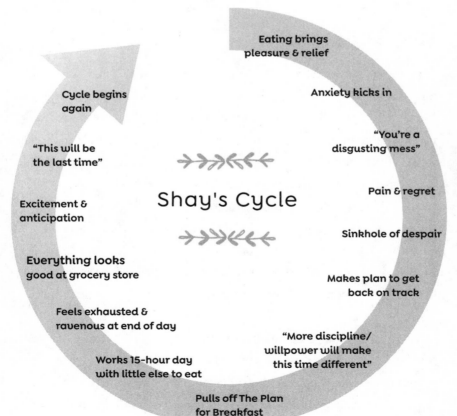

Cycle begins again

Eating brings pleasure & relief

Anxiety kicks in

"This will be the last time"

"You're a disgusting mess"

Excitement & anticipation

Shay's Cycle

Pain & regret

Everything looks good at grocery store

Sinkhole of despair

Feels exhausted & ravenous at end of day

Makes plan to get back on track

Works 15-hour day with little else to eat

"More discipline/ willpower will make this time different"

Pulls off The Plan for Breakfast

We wonder what it is like to read Shay's story and see her cycle laid out like this. Perhaps you already see parts of your own pattern in here. And if this doesn't quite fit for you, keep reading. In this next section, we take a closer look at different parts of The Cycle so you can begin to understand how it operates in your life. The predictable stages we explore include The Problem, The Surrounds, The Shame Shitstorm, The Plan, and Life, before it ultimately repeats.

The Problem

The best place to start determining your own cycle is by naming the thing you do with food that you wish you would "just stop already or get over." Most people have called this The Problem. Much like Shay and others who have come through our doors, this is most often identified as:

Emotional eating

Overeating

Eating "bad" things

Binge eating

Jen and Eva thought any eating was the problem. Shay told us she had a very clear idea about what she should be eating and how much she should be exercising to feel like she was "on track." But a few times a week she'd find herself unable to stop eating after work. She'd sometimes head to the store on her way home to buy her favorite "forbidden" foods, the ones she couldn't stop thinking about. Every time she thought, "This will be the last time." And yet, through all her effort to eradicate this behavior, she'd never found something to stop it from happening. She was confused because it caused her so much pain and regret.

Here are some questions to explore The Problem:

✳   What eating do you do that you are most judgmental about?

✳   When do you feel most out of control with your eating?

✳   Diet culture tends to label certain types of food or ways of eating as problematic. How do you judge your own eating through the lens of diet culture?

The Surrounds

The Surrounds are all the thoughts, feelings, and behaviors, as well as cultural instruction and validation, that lead up to or happen at the same time as The Problem. It might be how you have prepared for a binge or the sequence of events that led up to emotional eating. These thoughts, feelings, behaviors, and reactions may be overshadowed by the frustration about The Problem, but they are an important part of the puzzle.

The Surrounds includes how you feel and what you experience when engaging in The Problem. Some people hate this part and dissociate or numb out for the entire event. Others, like Shay, say that before they eat they often feel "rebellious and pissed off" and describe how exciting it is to round up the food they are going to eat. The excitement that occurs with the anticipation of eating all these forbidden foods brings some relief and is often the very best part. Shay shared that when she begins to eat the food she's gathered, she initially enjoys the flavors and textures. It's like a big exhale. There is a reward here. But soon after she starts eating, she notices a running dialogue of anxiety and judgment in her head. The more she eats, the more checked out she feels. She says she never feels done eating, and because she experiences shame while she eats, she "knows it's emotional eating." Shay is not yet able to see how trying to be good—the deprivation and restraint—gives rise to the eating she is judging.

Here are a few questions to think about to help bring clarity to this part of the cycle:

* What was happening before you found yourself engaging in The Problem? What were you doing? How were you feeling? What were you thinking?

* How do you feel when you are engaging in The Problem? What else is happening?

* What are you getting from the behavior? How does it help? What are the rewards, no matter how short-lived?

* What is it actually like to eat the food? Yummy? Scary? Fun? Relieving? Numbing? All of the above?

* What's your eating been like in the hours and days leading up to The Problem? Have you been eating regularly throughout the day, or skipping meals?

The Shame Shitstorm

After The Problem occurs, it is common for folks to descend into what we have come to call The Shame Shitstorm. Why is it called this?

It feels like hell.

This is the place where we feel regret, frustration, and hopelessness about what has happened. It is where the inner critic is shouting from a pedestal and the center of our being becomes flooded with shame. In the middle of the storm we hear:

> *You are disgusting.*
>
> *You are undisciplined.*
>
> *Why can't you get it together?*
>
> *What's wrong with you?*

And we feel . . .

Hot burning shame

Disgust

Self-rejection

Fear, sometimes incredibly intense fear

Self-loathing

Hopelessness

Frustration

Anger

Trapped or stuck

When Shay started to describe this part of her cycle she said, "Ugh, this part is the worst." You could see her demeanor shift as she descends into an all-too-familiar sinkhole of despair. The disappointment in herself was overwhelming. The imposter in her was terrified this is all she is. She had visions of being "better behaved" but could never seem to "pull it off." She was unbelievably frustrated. When we look at Jen's body story in the beginning of this chapter, this is where she felt it was easier not to listen to or feel hunger and connect to her needs.

In all of this, the biggest challenge is that we are afraid this shame pit represents who we really are. That this is our "true" self and the rest of the time we are just fooling people. These moments validate everything we have ever ingested from the world that said doubt her, they're untrustworthy, he is not enough. Our imposter complex is born from here. And without some resilience to This Shame Shit-storm, things can become paradoxical—because we end up needing the cycle more than ever.

Here are some questions to explore The Shame Shitstorm:

*   What thoughts and feelings arise after The Problem occurs? What do you say to yourself?

*   How do you know when you feel shame? What do you feel? What do you think?

*   What does The Shame Shitstorm look and sound like in your body/your life?

The Plan

Just like a knight on a white horse (which no one ever needed), The Plan comes swooping in to rescue us from the mucky, tar-like pit of shame and despair. The Plan (much like the knight, right?) is of the culture. It's the ideas, schedules, rules, and beliefs offered from the external world to "rescue you" from your whole intact divine self. Full of false promises, The Plan feels like it can make you into the ideal you: shame-proof, protected and fantastic, worthy of love, respect, and belonging. But just like that damn knight, it's full of empty promises, false fronts, ego, and lies.

You know the plans we're talking about, right? The Plan could be anything from a mainstream popular diet program (or the I-swear-this-isn't-a-diet diet), 30-day reset plan, intermittent fasting, a cleanse, another gym membership, cutting out this and giving up that. These plans ignite an uplifting promise of becoming better, less messy, more together, smaller, and successful at the thing that has most eluded you. When these plans swoop in to rescue us, it doesn't seem to matter if we've done them before and they haven't been sustainable or if they come with warning labels. We have been conditioned to believe in what they offer and we are desperate for an end to The Shame Shitstorm.

"Having a Plan is initially a huge relief," said Shay. It pulled her up and out of the deep well of shame and put her back in her head, where she felt more in control, distanced from difficult emotions, and less like a failure. She'd tried everything from a commercial diet plan to a 30-day "clean eating" program, a cleanse, or a work out plan, and although nothing worked, it felt better to believe more discipline, more willpower, and more organization would make this time different.

Here's the thing. We never blame The Plan. We have learned to blame ourselves, internalizing failure and self-doubt over and over again. This is a certainty because, as we discuss throughout this book, these plans do not work for the majority of people. Our bodies have strong physiological and psychological responses to food restriction and dietary restraint. We become preoccupied with food, which creates a feeling of being obsessed and "addicted." We get further distanced from hunger and fullness cues, as well as other somatic signals that help us make decisions about our nourishment. Our metabolism is impacted by food deprivation, a long-term impact for short-term gain. Our bodies do not know about dieting, they just know there isn't enough food being consumed to meet our needs and they create cravings and preoccupation with food to defend homeostasis for survival.

We want you to know that it is common for people to lose their tolerance to food deprivation and dietary restriction over time. The plans you made at the beginning of your quest for change may have lasted a lot longer than they do now. By the time folks arrive on the Body Trust doorstep, their plans are sustained for just a couple of minutes to a few days. The culture might call this a sign of poor discipline or a lack of willpower or tell you that you just haven't found the right plan. We see it as a sign of well-being and health. You see, our bodies are wired to survive famine— they don't like dieting—and yet nobody ever thinks to call the food restriction, restrained eating, or weight cycling the problem.

The real problem is the supremacy and dominance in our culture that has equated status with the pursuit of health (i.e., thinness) while diminishing key contributors to ill health—oppression, trauma, stigma, discrimination, and social location.

Here are some questions to explore The Plan:

* What would be different for you if you blamed The Plan instead of yourself?

* How is it for you to consider that these plans have never truly been sustainable?

* What would shift if you started to see food restriction and restrained eating as The Problem?

* What is one thing you do not want to forget from this section about The Plan?

Life

Let's be clear, real life is complicated and messy at times. (At the time of writing this, we are in year two of a global pandemic!) We fall in and out of love, struggle with finances, manage changes in housing, relationships, money, love. We live in bodies categorized in a hierarchy of perceived value, rooted in upholding white-thin-cis-het-abled identity as the most normative and ideal. Size is one of the markers that often falsely signals less worthiness. Our needs change, our wants change, our bodies change, and so do all the people around us. Real lives are messy, inherently. They are not truly controllable. Just like the people in the stories we have shared in this chapter, we have punished and judged ourselves for our life messes and twists and turns. Instead of knowing the ups and downs of our lives are normal—to be expected—and not a measure of our worthiness, we assess our worth by how together we have it. Having it all together (which is a way perfectionism expresses itself) begins to become congruent with other measures of status handed to us by the dominant culture like thinness and muscle tone, athleticism, wealth, partnerships, etc. The list goes on and on. And none of this is the reason we are alive. None of this is what we came here to do.

Shay was surprised when we asked her about this part. She had assumed life should never get in the way of her success with The Plan because everyone knows you are supposed to make it work despite life. She'd get mad at herself when life got too "lifey" (thanks to Anne Lamott for this term!) and she'd "blow it with food." But she also acknowledged that her job was busy and variable—she was working up to sixty hours a week sometimes—and travel was often involved. She's the go-to in her community for support and was always the one to show up with food or start the GoFundMe for folks in need. She was responsible for coordinating care for her mother with Alzheimer's, and she was the backup care provider for her nephew whenever her brother needed help.

Shay was taught by popular culture to see her care for others as getting in the way of prioritizing her plans, and this overly individualized focus is always the priority in diet culture. The culture does not validate the truth: relational connections and commitments are often not optional or "in the way." Shay was surprised when we asked her if she believed the relentless pursuit of thinness via "perfect eating" had made her healthy. Would she be healthier with less connection in her life? This reframe was brand-new for her.

Here are some questions to explore this stage of The Cycle:

* What are some of the ways perfectionism colors the way you experience your life?

* How has diet culture encouraged you to prioritize The Plan over other core values in your life?

* What expectations do you have for yourself that get in the way of your finding joy and pleasure in life?

Closing the Loop

You may already have a clear sense of what closes the loop and returns us to our familiar coping pattern (and what we have called The Problem). Engaging repeatedly in this cycle requires a lot of effort and planning. It contains a lot of feelings. It fuels disappointment, frustration, shame, and self-harm. The Cycle itself creates the need for coping.

Human beings have a remarkable ability to make things harder than they need to be, especially when feeling anxious or stressed, flooded with shame, or powerless or alone. When we are frustrated with the way life is or the way we handle our lives, we tend to pull in the reins, raising the expectations and the stakes.

What we really need is spaciousness and room to breathe, feel, and center ourselves again. But because slowing down is hard when our nervous systems are amped up, and we aren't practiced at trusting a slowdown, we often reach for coping in all of its predictable, dissociative numbness. Uncomfortably comfortable and all-too-familiar. For many people, this is the most accessible way to keep going in a world that wasn't made for them.

Shay spoke to how anxious she felt in this part of the cycle. With more awareness, she began to notice that when her plan was disrupted, she became more fearful, judgmental, and hopeless. She'd make more (ultimately meaningless) rules to punish herself *and* as a last-ditch effort to stop herself from engaging in The Problem again. She wished there were better answers. She was surprised to hear she's not alone. She started to understand how this coping has been wise, and that maybe this struggle really wasn't her fault.

Here are a few more questions for you:

* What are the expectations you hold for yourself that feel like you will never measure up to?

* What are some of the ways you are beginning to see the wisdom in your coping?

* If you could go back in time and tell your younger self about your experiences with diet culture (or disordered eating), what would you want them to know? What would you warn them about?

Illuminating Your Pattern of Coping You Developed to Survive

One thing we know for sure is this: it is hard to disrupt the pattern or shift the cycle when you are not aware of it, when you cannot see it. In her book *Don't Let It Get You Down*, Savala Nolan, who is mixed race, writes:

> *I'm fat in ways that my white mom didn't understand, and still doesn't; nearing eighty, she diets and rebels, diets and rebels, still trapped in the cycle of perfecting, or at least improving, her body, still riding the cycle's restrictions and hopes and the impending fall off the wagon. When she sleeps at our house, she sometimes waits until the lights are out, then pads to the kitchen and eats more, leaning alone against the counter. At Thanksgiving, the table in candlelight, she says, "Starting tomorrow, no more sugar and no more junk." These are things I have done too. She is my mom; I wish she were free.[1]*

Every chapter in this book holds a possibility, a clue, or a practice to help you learn more about and begin shifting your cycle so you can move more deeply into this work. You'll discover where shame lives and how it functions in the cycle, and where restriction lies (shame and restriction are almost always at play in the cycle, no matter what you call The Problem: your body, your food choices, overeating, emotional eating, etc.).

Eva was surprised to see what her cycle looked like as a complete picture. And like most folks we work with, she was eager to find a way out. Eva said:

It started with me rejecting my body by trying to hide and run away. So now, as I've come to terms with what I see in the mirror, I say it doesn't have to be a way to hide anymore. It doesn't have to be a way to reject the rest of the world. Let who I am be. I don't wanna have to fix myself over and over to be okay, acceptable. I can like myself as I am. The depth of the layers of it are unexpected.

Eva's story reminds us that healing is a process, not a destination, and that this work is about creating a relationship with ourselves that isn't reliant on us staying any one way.

Begin by naming your cycle. As you investigate, familiarize yourself with the chaining of thoughts, feelings, sensations, and behaviors that arise in the pattern, as well as how other people in your life intersect with it. Get curious about what happens next and then what. What do your plans sound like? What is happening in your life just before you end up in The Problem again? Widen the lens: Is what you are calling The Problem really the problem? Might the problem be that you are not regularly getting enough to eat? When you are in the beginning stages of recognizing how this cycle works through you, there are a few places to practice doing things differently right away.

Making a Plan for No Plan

One of the first places people catch themselves in The Cycle is in the planning, and the best way to disrupt the cycle is to resist the urge to make a plan. Essentially, when you notice yourself in planning mode, ask yourself, as coach Sam Dylan Finch wrote in an Instagram post, "Do I want to go another round, or do I want to turn this around?" It doesn't feel so simple internally, because what we are choosing is far more layered, as Eva said. Compassionately, we are saying, "I trust myself to try a new pattern today. I trust myself to try and withstand something different. I trust my early coping and I trust how my coping can evolve. I can see that this pattern is no longer who I am. I want to express something new."

We want you to try life without a plan.* Is this scary? We guess yes. Is it dangerous? No, it is not. Remember you, your food, and your body are not a problem to be solved. Adopt a phrase you can repeat to yourself when you are feeling pulled to make a plan. Something like "My plan is for no plan." Or "No fixin' No fixin' No fixin'." Or "My plan is for radical self-preservation."

What is radical self-preservation? It is a kind of self-care that nourishes your sense of worthiness and isn't tied to changing the size of your body. It is what Durryle Brooks describes as "ways of being, knowing, orienting, and acting that help reconstitute the very core of who I am," moving "from a place of performative self-care to the set of practices that made me feel whole and most like myself."[2] Here's one of our favorite questions to ask folks in our workshops, retreats, and trainings:

If you woke up tomorrow and lived in a body-affirming, weight-inclusive world where you regularly experienced love, respect, and belonging, what would you do to care for yourself? What would you suddenly have permission to do more of? Less of?

Let your answers be a guidepost.

Redefine What Healing Looks and Feels Like

When people start exploring Body Trust, they often think, "It's not working," meaning "I'm not losing weight" or "I'm still eating sugar/emotionally eating/bingeing, so I must be doing something wrong." Shifting away from diet culture's view of progress means our intentions and hopes become more personal and less oriented toward perfecting

---

* We know many readers are in the process of recovering from an eating disorder and are relying on their meal plan as a part of their healing process. This is not the type of plan we are referring to. We invite you to discern: Is my plan moving me toward something that supports the entirety of my well-being? We encourage you to discuss this with your treatment providers (if applicable) or someone who knows the history of your eating disorder and has your best interest in mind.

food and our bodies. This requires you to put aside thoughts about weight/nutrition/health so you can develop compassionate, weight-neutral practices that are connected to your needs and desires, flexible and forgiving (as opposed to rigid and perfectionistic) and more pleasurable and satisfying.

Most of the people we've worked with over the years have been coping with food for so long that it is understandable—and expected—that you will continue your patterns at the same time you are unraveling and unhooking from them. Patterns and behaviors are not usually the first thing to change in the process of reclaiming body trust, which is why we encourage you to begin by redefining what healing looks and feels like for you.

In the reckoning phase of this healing work, people often consider the possibility of change for a much longer period of time than they actually act on change. So expect that even while you are healing and growing, you will lean on familiar ways to cope in the same way you always have. Remember, it's a foundation of Body Trust to honor this expression of self-preservation. You may notice a shift in the frequency and severity of certain behaviors. Abstinence is not the goal here.

The question is, what would it be like to accept that the behaviors you are trying to change are in fact going to happen sometimes? That this is a part of how you have survived and you will continue to rely on this to get through the change process? Is it possible to have some gratitude for this wise form of coping, even if you also find it tiresome or frustrating? Can you accept that you are in process and this cycle has been an integral part of who you have become?

Depending on how long you've had a challenging relationship with food and your body, this cycle can be deeply grooved or fairly shallow. Once you are more familiar with your pattern, you will start to notice when you are being hijacked by it. It is through this awareness that you can start to disrupt the cycle and find various ways to shift, change, loosen the grip, and ultimately transform it.

Look and Listen with Kindness and Curiosity

A final reminder: be gentle with yourself. Judgment, as well as our inner critic, have a way of spinning a single narrow narrative about our lived experience. They shut down curiosity, which is necessary for change. As we discussed in The Foundations section, curiosity, coupled with kindness, creates an opening to witness your inner workings with fresh eyes. What you may see, as you watch and learn from your own cycle, may provide you with the very information and insight needed to support the change you are seeking. Jen Inaldo speaks to this in her body story:

> *My body is this nebulous thing. Sometimes I consciously avoid going too deeply; its mysterious rolling hills and valleys and dark places scare me. Knowing what lies beneath this skin means knowing everything.*
>
> *It's easier to move through this world a bag of spaghetti and bones, inconsequential and tangible and easy to swallow. Not this dark sticky confusing mass of secrets.*
>
> *What if I look closely and confirm:*
>
> *There is nothing special here. You are not worth knowing.*
>
> *I can't look at my round calves and proclaim their greatness. I can't present to you my belly, separated into two hemispheres, my belly button living in the deep fold of my equator, and tell you that this is love.*
>
> *The most I can spare is two long minutes in front of the bathroom mirror upon first waking up. My hair sticks straight up and out of the messy bun I slept in, reaching for the sky. This is okay.*
>
> *My face with fresh lines telling me I slept hard last night. This is okay.*
>
> *I wipe the crust from my eyes and adjust my glasses and look again.*
>
> *This is what I look like. This is what I look like.*

This is how I love you. This is how I love you.

Again and again. It has to start small. Everything else may or may not come along for the ride, but today this is enough and I wash my face with cold water and my dog finds me and licks my calves, telling me he is ready to start the day.

We are aware you may want to skip ahead. We know how uncomfortable it can be to sit with what is and not have all of the answers. We encourage you to pause, slow down, and give yourself a chance to lean into the questions and learn more about the unique ways the various stages of The Cycle show up in your life. You deserve to know. And the information revealed will help you in your healing and liberation. We promise the time spent will be worth it, as Maya G., a Body Trust program participant, said:

> *This is an endless cycle, and it doesn't work. You will lose and gain the same thirty to fifty pounds over and over again. You will get a vision of yourself as a thinner person, you will plan a diet and/or exercise program, you will start the program, you will get hungry and immediately stop the program, YOU WILL EAT, and then you will feel guilty and start to plan another diet. Or you will maintain your commitment for a certain period of time, lose some weight, and then gain it back. You might even gain more, because your body was starving and now it's holding on to the weight. You will blame yourself, your lack of willpower, and feel hatred toward your body and self.*
>
> *There's another way, and it's not about trying harder; it's about trying something different. You can learn to trust your body to tell you what it wants and needs. You can learn to trust there will always be more delicious food, and you don't need to eat everything right now. You can learn that diets are designed to fail so you keep coming back, and the only trustworthy thing is healing your relationship to food and your*

body. It will take time to integrate new ways of seeing food, exercise, and your body as a trustworthy being. It will be worth it. I promise.

The webpage for the readers of this book offers a variety of resources, worksheets, and guided meditations to learn how The Cycle operates in your unique life.

 ## ANNA'S BODY STORY

I remember seeing lots of low-fat commercials the summer I realized my body was headed to fat town. In my family, fat town was not a place we visited, nor were we allowed to have any peace when we arrived. I remember when I sized out of Ross Dress for Less before they really had a plus area. I cried in the dressing room because I saw the pain in my mom's eyes. Before this, I relished feeding my body, and my love for food was pure. After this, my body was no longer mine, it was a disappointment, and if I had any hope of salvaging my life as a tenish-year-old I needed to get it together.

I often looked to my mom for how to feel after I lost my body to her disappointment. I stopped understanding hunger cues and gave up choice. If I was being a GOOD little GURL, I was eating small portions, no snacks, kept a journal of every morsel that entered my mouth, and would go on walks with my parents for the bare minimum thirty minutes of huff and puff (a terrible term coined by the world's worst child dietitian). Not play or joyful movement. Walks. (News flash: Kids don't give a shit about exercise and walks are boring.) There was peace in my house, and everyone was super proud of me. But when I eventually restricted one too many cookies as a preteen, I would go rogue and be a

BAD little GURL. I would fucking rage, taking small sums of cash from my mom's wallet to buy candy at the pro shop after swim practice. I would run to the kitchen and take lightning-speed scoops of ice cream and run them to my room. I was so tired of not being allowed to want, and this was a spiteful way to get back at my mom for being disappointed in me. I was in a constant state of scarcity, fearing my last desirable food would be taken away and in its place nothing but bell peppers and homemade hummus would remain.

For over fifteen years, the only thing that mattered was getting thin. I wasn't able to make a meal, take a walk, buy an outfit, or even kiss a person without thinking about how disappointing my body was. How being fat was the worst thing that could ever happen to me. One day in therapy, I heard myself say, "Until I'm thin I won't be loved, I won't get married, I won't have a good job, a nice car, or the clothes that I want," and something in me broke open. My heart heard the lie and something came alive in me. I read books, I found fat friends, I bought a dress that was made for my body. I ate the whole cake and realized that I could eat cake every day . . . and then I moved on to ice cream. There was a permission happening that was more of a longing to be free than a broken-down will. My willpower shifted from starving me to wanting the previously impossible . . . freedom to exist without hating my body.

I had to come out as fat. It was weird and I thought it was obvious. But what I found was that coming out was more for me than anyone else. I had to meet my mom and the disappointment I thought she held over me my whole life. I had to meet my own self-loathing. I had to meet my internalized hate for my fat community and see that I was falsely taught to hate my body. I had done nothing wrong by being fat, and neither had any other fat person. I actually learned that hating my body and starving it contributed to making it more fat!

So where is she now, you might be asking yourselves?

I've dedicated my life to supporting my fat community in knowing they are valuable and wonderful lights in our society. I'm a fat activist who works in the movement, wellness, and fashion industry to fight for our rights to be served with as many options and tools as folks in smaller bodies receive. I have found people to date who celebrate my fat body right along with me. And let me just clear something up, until I started to heal my internalized fatphobia (it's a lifelong process that I'm not sure I'll ever be completely healed from), I didn't get all of those things I longed for. But today in 2021, I have a thriving career, a perfect angel companion dog, a big nice car, and the clothes I once dreamed of . . . all while living in my super fat body.

Now isn't that some shit? My advice to you is to do what you want, seek freedom, and stop lamenting a body that was never here for you. Your body is waiting to live its fullest life with you, no matter the make or model. Keep going, angels, it gets better.

Part II

The Reckoning

We just explored how you lost trust with your body. Now it's time for reckoning. We reckon when it becomes clear that something is no longer serving us. We think and feel into what changes this healing process will bring and how that will be for us. We consider what we will gain, what we will lose. And we make our way through this reckoning by reading, listening, asking questions, overthinking, wishing, and grieving. Reckoning is a place of emotional honesty. You may feel anger, loss, and uncertainty, and you'll return, again and again, to wondering how you ended up here in the first place. As a result of this, your body story emerges with more clarity and becomes wholly yours. We reckon on our path to reclamation.

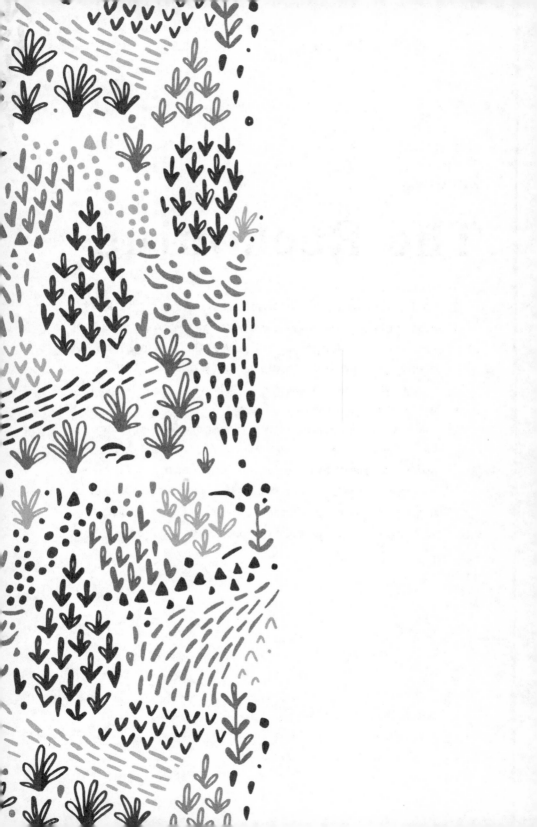

CHAPTER 4

Divesting from Diet Culture

Me claiming my ugliness does not mean I am claiming to be the opposite of beautiful. I am claiming freedom from anti-Black standards of beauty, from ableism, fatphobia, classism, the patriarchy and all the ways they have and continue to colonize our beautiful and majestic bodies, lives, and possibilities.[1]

—VANESSA ROCHELLE LEWIS, founding director of Reclaim Ugly

Many of the people we work with believe they gave up dieting years ago and that they've just been "watching what they are eating" or "trying to eat healthier" only to discover their efforts have still been rooted or invested in diet culture. When people come to explore Body Trust, they've maybe reckoned with the reality that diets don't work for them (and the majority of us), but they haven't returned to body trust. They've usually found new rationales and new plans to continue with dieting behaviors while calling it something else, like a healthy lifestyle, a cleanse, or intermittent fasting.

Diet culture is a sneaky shape-shifter. The weight loss, wellness, and cosmetic fitness industries know that "diet" is a four-letter word, so they co-opt anti-diet language and body positive phrasing while doing next to nothing to change their programs or offer something truly different. They are constantly repackaging their services while continuing to collude with oppressive and mechanistic ways of thinking about and inhabiting the body. They encourage you to hold on to the belief that if you just find the right program or the right way, everything will fall into place and a better version of you will be revealed to the world.

Noom is the latest we're-not-a-diet-it's-a-lifestyle diet. A mailer Dana received says "Let Noom open your mind to a new way to lose weight" and claims "psychologists are involved in the program to help you build healthy, lasting change." Their website says, "There are no good and bad foods, just green, yellow and red based on caloric content," inspired by a weight loss program for children called the Stoplight Diet. Instead of WW (Weight Watcher) points or calorie counting, people learn a new way to track and judge their choices based on yet another set of external guidelines. This categorization of foods just creates more noise in the brain and fuels rigid thoughts and food policing. It is highly unlikely that someone doing Noom is going to see a "red" food and not think it's a "bad" food. You know that phrase: If it looks like a duck, swims like a duck, and quacks like a duck, then it probably is a duck. Without a critical analysis of diet culture, it's easy to see why people buy into it.

Our socialization and indoctrination is so deep that we don't even think to question how we navigate the world of food, eating, and exercise. What we learn at home, in school, from health care providers, and society is taken as the truth, the word, the gospel. By the time doctors enter medical school, most have already made up their minds about fatness and health, and their training does little to challenge these deeply held beliefs. None of us are offered an opportunity for informed consent—a chance to fully understand the risks associated with food restriction and dietary restraint—before we start participating. As the years go by, our plans morph and change, but they are still rooted in a dieting mindset. When we develop a more critical lens, we start to see all the ways we are still invested in diet culture:

* Tying your worth to your weight, your looks, or your behaviors

* Seeking advice from outside "experts" to tell you what, when, and how much to eat/exercise

* Exercising primarily for the purpose of burning calories, controlling weight, cosmetic fitness

* Referencing calories, points, macros, etc., to determine what you will eat

* Judging a day of behaviors as good or bad

* Thinking about food in dichotomous terms like healthy/ unhealthy, clean/junk, right/wrong

* Putting up false food fronts, where you ignore your own needs and desires to perform health when you are with people

* Using fitness apps to determine how you are doing with that calories in/calories out equation

* Keeping your smaller clothes with the intention of fitting back into them some day

* Being preoccupied with healthy eating or identifying "nutrition, health, and wellness" as a hobby

* Weighing, measuring, tracking, monitoring, scrutinizing

* Suppressing your natural weight despite your body's repeated attempts to return to where it is comfortable

* Upholding and complimenting weight loss

*   Pedestaling people who appear to have it all together with their willpower/discipline/control

*   Making disparaging comments about fat people

*   Talking about celebrity eating habits, food/fitness plans, etc., with others

*   Restricting and restraining your food followed by rebellious or backlash eating (cheat days)

*   Experiencing shame after you eat some foods and feeling pride when you eat others

*   Believing in willpower

*   Creating a plan for how you are going to "make up" for your choices

*   Thinking it's "not working" or "not worth it" if your body isn't changing

*   Defining success by the number on the scale or the size of your clothes/body

After reading through this list, you may feel surprised and even a little defensive if you've never considered how this way of thinking is harmful and problematic, both to you and to society at large. This mentality is part of a culture that upholds thinness under the guise of health and believes health is the *be-all and end-all* to our existence. We cannot fathom that it is possible to be fat and healthy (despite the evidence available but rarely discussed), so those of us who are not actively pursuing health (and thinness) by engaging with food and our bodies in this performative way are viewed as in denial, lacking discipline and self-control. And the fatter you are, the more unworthy you are of love, respect, and belonging. It is no wonder The Hustle continues.

When we look at health through a wider lens to include health equity and social justice, research consistently shows that the social determinants of health have a far greater impact on our health and well-being than our weight or individual lifestyle behaviors. These determinants include all forms of stigma and oppression as well as social, economic, and environmental factors like access to a living wage, nutritious food, clean air and water, stable housing, childcare, reproductive justice, health care, and more. We appreciate this image by Holisticallygrace that illustrates what we ignore when we have a myopic focus on diet and exercise.

The Health Iceberg

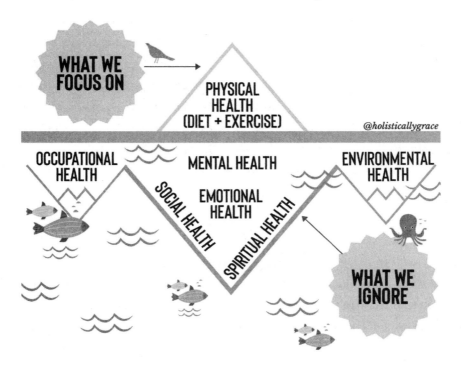

Here's one example: You may have heard about the health benefits of eating a Mediterranean diet rich in fruits and nuts, vegetables, legumes, whole grains, and healthy fats. In 2017, a study with over 18,000

subjects published in the *International Journal of Epidemiology* found that "The Mediterranean diet reduces the risk of cardiovascular disease but only if you are rich or highly educated."[2] So basically, if you have a lower socioeconomic status but eat a Mediterranean diet, it has little impact on your heart health. We need more researchers asking questions like this to help us adequately look at and understand the complex set of factors that impact the health of an individual as well as the communities in which they live. Radical dietitian and poet Lucy Aphramor once said (in a Health at Every Size training), "You can tell a lot more about a person's health by looking at their ZIP code than their BMI."

If we deeply care about health—our own as well as others—and want to help improve the health of the population at large, our time, money, and energy would be better spent doing anti-oppression work and fighting for social justice than telling people to eat healthier, take a bubble bath, try intermittent fasting, or exercise to manage their weight. But people treat wellness like a religion, and when they discover a new product, program, or plan that "works" in the short term (i.e., weight loss or food control), they love to convert others to their mission, particularly when they are in the "honeymoon phase" of the plan. Meanwhile, oppressive systems continue to impact people's lives in much more significant and profound ways.

The culture spouts off about the importance of living a healthy lifestyle and the medical industrial complex leans on personal responsibility rhetoric, all while ignoring and/or doing little to address the social determinants of health. A few years ago, our DEI (diversity, equity, and inclusion) consultant Jessica Fish asked a group of us at a retreat, "What if the kind of care we are advocating for isn't a form of self-care but rather a form of divestment?" To divest means to dig up the roots. When we begin divesting from diet culture, we must root out the ways we have been conditioned to think about size, beauty, health, and weight. As we dig into our body stories, we are considering how we became so aware of and invested in controlling and perfecting food and our bodies. We did not consent to this mindset. Our participation has not necessarily been deeply connected to our wisest self. And many of us continue to believe this is the only way to occupy and care for a body when our lived experience tells us, over and over again, just how difficult it is to pull off long term. Becoming more aware of these beliefs and investigating their origins in systemic oppression while learning more about Body Trust will give you a chance to decide what you truly believe, what you want to hold on to (if anything), and what was never yours to embody that you now want to let go of.

Desiree Adaway, founder and principal of The Adaway Group, created The Praxis for Liberation from the steps she's cultivated in her life for getting free. She says:

> We defy the lies we have been told. We defend the truth. We demand transformation (of ourselves and the world!). We declare our nonnegotiables for Freedom and divest from chains that hold us down and hold us back. We dream together.

Before we can defy the lies, we need to know the truth about bodies, food, weight, and health, since our socialization and the toxic atmosphere in which we live make it impossible to see. So what is the truth we are defending?

* Bodies have existed across a diverse spectrum of presentations since the beginning of time, and there's no one right way to have a body.

* Human metabolism is far more complex than a "calories in/calories out" equation.

* Health is as diverse and complex as bodies themselves and exists on a continuum from the moment we are conceived in the womb until we take our last breath.

* Health is not attainable for some people and never will be. Despite popular rhetoric, every health condition cannot and will not be cured through diet and lifestyle.

* Trauma, oppression (i.e., racism, weight stigma), and eating disorders have much more significant impacts on a person's health than their weight or lifestyle choices.

* We have less control over many things in our lives than we'd like to believe, including our weight and our health.

* A complex set of physiological factors kick in after weight loss occurs, making maintenance of a lower body weight difficult for all but a small minority.

* Food is deeply personal. It's flavored with meaning. Food connects us to our history, our culture, our ancestors, our religion, our traditions. When we mess with our food, we are messing with our sense of who we are—our identity—in ways we rarely anticipate or understand.

* There's no one right way to eat for everybody, and the next fad diet is right around the corner waiting to throw the current one under the bus.

* One day of eating does not have the power to make you gain or lose weight, nor does it have the power to suddenly make you healthy or unhealthy. (We're not talking about things like peanut allergies here!) In terms of lifestyle choices, bodies are most impacted by what we do repeatedly and consistently over significant periods of time.

* You cannot look at someone and know what their food and exercise behaviors are and whether or not they are healthy.

* The body mass index (BMI) has racist roots. It is being
  misused to stigmatize and pathologize bodies and is not
  evidence based.

In recent years, more and more has been written about the problematic origins of the BMI. In an essay titled "A Brief History of the Fat
Acceptance Movement," Sirius Bonner writes,

> *Anti-fat bias and fat-phobia are deeply rooted in white suprem-
> acy and anti-blackness.* Sabrina Strings's book Fearing the
> Black Body: The Racial Origins of Fat Phobia *argues that as color
> became more complicated because of rape and miscegenation
> in early America, body size became another way of understand-
> ing who was enslaved and who was not, and, by extension,
> who was Black and who was white. This product of white su-
> premacy became intertwined with the deeply patriarchal pro-
> ject of keeping women literally and figuratively small. This put
> white women in the position of having to remain slender in or-
> der to recoup the benefits of correctly performing their gender
> and race. Further, this early period solidified cultural associa-
> tions between laziness, fatness, and Blackness which have car-
> ried through mostly unchanged to the current day.*

In the nineteenth century, the BMI was developed by Belgian stat-
istician Adolphe Quetelet to look at the distribution of weight across
a population of white people. It was never created for, nor intended to
be used on, individuals to determine health status; but since the 1970s,
doctors' offices, insurance companies, and government statisticians have
relied on it to assess fatness and fitness. In her 2019 *Medium* article,
"The Bizarre and Racist History of the BMI," Aubrey Gordon writes:

> *Quetelet believed that the mathematical mean of a popula-
> tion was its ideal, and his desire to prove it resulted in the
> invention of the BMI, a way of quantifying* l'homme moyen's

[the average man's] weight. Initially called Quetelet's Index, [the formula was] based solely on the size and measurements of French and Scottish participants. That is, the Index was devised exclusively by and for white Western Europeans. By the turn of the next century, Quetelet's l'homme moyen would be used as a measurement of fitness to parent, and as a scientific justification for eugenics—the systemic sterilization of disabled people, autistic people, immigrants, poor people, and people of color.[3]

The BMI and its uses have evolved over time. In the 1990s, BMI cutoffs were lowered arbitrarily (the American Medical Association did not support the change), which created an opportunity for pharmaceutical and weight loss companies to earn more money overnight. In their book *Body Respect*, Lindo Bacon and Lucy Aphramor debunk seven myths about fatness, including that BMI is a valuable and accurate health measure. They write:

Examine the international standards, set by the World Health Organization (WHO), and you will find that the WHO relied on the International Obesity Task Force (IOTF) to make the recommendations. At the time, the two biggest funders of the IOTF were the pharmaceutical companies that had the only weight loss drugs on the market. In other words, the pharmaceutical industry which has a vested interest in making us believe that fat is dangerous—and that they have a solution— wrote the BMI standards that are currently used. The derivation of children's BMI standards was even worse. They were just arbitrarily assigned, without even the pretense of considering health data. The facts show that many people in the BMI categories of "overweight" and "obese" live long, disease-free lives. In other words, fatness alone doesn't mean sickness. Other measures of fatness, including hydrostatic weighing and bioelectric impedance, waist-hip ratio and waist circumference, are similarly flawed.[4]

In addition to understanding the problematic history of the BMI, we find plenty to critique about the field of "obesity medicine and weight science" fueled by rampant anti-fat bias, flawed data, and a crisis of imagination. It's rare for studies reporting correlations between weight and health to control for things like socioeconomic status, stress from discrimination, weight cycling, fitness levels, and use of weight loss drugs, all of which have an impact on health outcomes. Correlation is not the same thing as causation. The way the medical community is using the BMI to categorize our bodies into under-, normal, overweight, and obese categories impacts the kind of care we receive, our eligibility and premiums for insurance, and our access to lifesaving surgeries and medical treatment.

Even if, after reading all this, you still believe that being fat is bad for your health and people should keep trying to lose, then what is the evidence-based treatment for high body weight that leads to sustained weight loss? There isn't a single program that has five-year outcome data to support it, and yet health care providers keep recommending weight loss when the data and their clinical experience show the most consistent effect of weight loss at two years is weight gain.[5,6] It seems our bodies have a place where they are comfortable weight-wise, and we can spend our entire lives trying to suppress our natural weight (and likely weight cycling, which research shows has harmful impacts on health)—or we can come to terms with reality, move on with our lives, find new ways of caring for ourselves that aren't rooted in shame and disembodiment, and trust our bodies to sort out our weight.

Years ago, someone made a comment on one of Dana's social media posts about Body Trust and compared our work to that of climate change deniers. We know that the information we've just shared is not the science that gets touted in the media. It's not the science that gets research funding. It doesn't fuel a multibillion-dollar industry making money off our shame and fragmentation. Our education and training don't give us the tools to become critical viewers of the dominant weight paradigm. And we certainly do not learn how anti-fatness and the body mass index are rooted in anti-Blackness.[7] Even when people are exposed to the truth, it's hard to reckon with. We keep chasing thin privilege and the illusion of control to avoid being othered. Choosing a different path rooted in our wholeness and our humanity (and our ethics, if we are helping professionals and health care providers) means we will be misunderstood, judged, rejected, and gaslit. The good news is there is a growing community of people doing the work to divest from diet culture.

In our process of divestment, it can be useful to begin thinking about beauty, health, fitness, weight, and gender as social constructs— "something that doesn't exist independently in the 'natural' world, but is instead an invention of society. Cultural practices and norms give rise to the existence of social constructs and govern practices, customs, and rules concerning the way we use/view/understand them."[8] These constructs restrict agency and impact the way we engage with the world by maintaining the status quo.

Let's first look at how beauty is socially constructed. When you ask young children what they find beautiful, their answers often don't match what adults say because of our socialization. Hilary's son's remarkable preschool teacher, Joe Bryan, asked his class "What is beautiful?" after noticing people's interest in defining beauty for his daughter. Throughout the school year, children were invited to bring what they found beautiful to class, filling walls and countertops, paper and projects. Their contributions were always included, never corrected or reframed, and were ever evolving. Parents were eventually invited to view this creative process and found dirt, mud, garbage, colors, layers, and life. Compiled beauty, related to in a moment, and then added to the fray and moved on from. Viewing this project challenged the adults' neater and tidier indoctrinated ideas of beauty, as what the children created was not recognizable as such immediately. This moment, in a preschool classroom, helped unravel beauty. We wonder where you might find beauty if your ideas about it weren't socially constructed.

Beauty is something our body knows, maybe often, before we do. And we have been marinating in dominant ideas of beauty that, at times, have overridden our bodies' simple attraction to this or that or that person. We should be angrier about our indoctrination into beauty that tells us what and who we should be attracted to. How many people, experiences, ideas, and creations have you bypassed due to this indoctrination? What have we missed out on in the process? When the embodied response says *yes*, it should not need to be further explained or understood.

The standards of beauty, while they have evolved and changed over time, have always been set by people in power, i.e., people who are white, cis, thin, straight, able-bodied, wealthy, and typically male. The rest of us subscribe to and uphold these standards without question and resist what Vanessa Rochelle Lewis, founder of Reclaim UGLY, calls "Uglification," which, she writes, "consists of personal and cultural beliefs, behaviors, practices, and laws that dehumanize people as ugly, undesirable, immoral, and unworthy. It feeds, maintains, and depends on oppression, such as lookism, racism, ableism, sexism, and homo, trans, fat, and xenophobia. Unchecked, it facilitates, normalizes, and validates hatred, childhood bullying, workplace exclusion, criminalization, medical neglect, violence, exploitation, and more."[9]

The targeting of some gender representations in very specific ways make resisting the lifelong hustle particularly challenging. We cannot talk about divesting from diet culture without looking at how the social construct of gender—the social and cultural interpretation of sex—intersects with it. In the book *A Clinician's Guide to Gender-Affirming Care*, Sand Chang defines gender training as "the rigid, pervasive messages that we receive from a young age about what it means to be a boy/man or girl/woman, including rules about appearance, behavior, emotional expression, preferences and dislikes, and ways of relating to others."[10]

Some of these messages encourage the relentless pursuit of beauty, thinness, and desirability. Sabrina Strings writes: "The fear of the imagined 'fat Black woman'[11] was created by racial and religious ideologies that have been used to both degrade Black women and discipline white women." The objectification of white women's bodies in advertising increased after white women in America were granted the right to vote in 1920. The first Miss America pageant took place in September of 1921. And then a drastic increase was observed when this objectification was problematized in the 1970s by feminist groups. In her book *The Beauty Myth*, Naomi Wolf writes: "A culture fixated on female thinness is not an obsession with female beauty, but an obsession with female obedience." She goes on to say, "Dieting is the most potent political sedative in women's history; a quietly mad population is a tractable one."[12] We believe this is one reason why 48 to 53 percent of white women voted for Mr. "Grab-em-by-the-pussy" in both the 2016 and 2020 election despite his disrespectful views of women being well documented on film, radio interviews, and the like. He's been accused of sexual assault by multiple women. And he was also the owner of the Miss Universe pageant from 1996 to 2015. In her memoir *Shrill*, Lindy West writes:

> *When you raise every woman to believe that we are insignificant, that we are broken, that we are sick, that the only cure is starvation and restraint and smallness; when you pit women against one another, keep us shackled by shame and hunger, obsessing over our flaws rather than our power and potential; when you leverage all of that to sap our money and our time— that moves the rudder of the world. It steers humanity toward conservatism and walls and the narrow interests of men, and it keeps us adrift in waters where women's safety and humanity are secondary to men's pleasure and convenience.*

A powerful shift occurs when we begin to think about who benefits when we are distracted by the relentless pursuit of thinness and beauty and desirability. The anger we've been directing internally starts to be externalized as we reckon with the ways we've been harmed and the ways we've upheld harm. We more clearly see what's been lost as we gain a critical analysis of social constructs.

The lack of analysis about the social construct of gender, or about the binary, linear, and polarized way our culture has constructed gender, creates harm. When one's gender identity does not match the sex assigned at birth, many but not all experience gender dysphoria, or clinically significant distress, and this can have significant impacts on the relationship with food and body. Trans people are over eight times more likely than cis women to have been diagnosed with an eating disorder.[13] On an episode of the Food Psych podcast,[14] Sand Chang talked about society's body norms for trans and nonbinary people and its layers in their own process of healing:

> There's a lot tied up with gender expression, sexuality, and how I was managing my appearance and weight ties into that because if I am at a smaller size, I may be seen as more masculine or more androgynous, whereas when I put on weight, maybe more curves, than I'm seen as a little bit more feminine. And for me it's not just how other people are seeing me, it's how I feel in my body as well . . . this idea that to be androgynous, you must really not have a body, it has to be totally neutral . . . the ideals we have for what trans bodies are supposed to look like are based on white, skinny, model-looking people and exclude folks who are fat, disabled, POC. There are so many ways in which these dominant norms and dominant representations of trans identity don't leave room for the vast majority of us.[15]

The way we think about health today is largely a social construct. When we look at the natural world, we know health exists on a continuum from the moment you are conceived in the womb until the moment you die. We know that not all bodies will have or maintain health.

That some will die in the womb, some will die young, some will have mobility issues, others will get cancer. Many will be able to reproduce, others not. Some will live relatively long lives with little to no health concerns until the ones associated with the natural aging process set in and they make their transition. How humans handle the reality of inhabiting a human body is socially constructed.

Since the 1980s, health has increasingly become a moral obligation, and people who aren't pursuing and performing health are viewed as morally inferior and less valuable. It has become common lore that if we just live a healthy lifestyle, we can control and have access to good health. While our behaviors and choices concerning lifestyle have some impact on our health and well-being, that impact is not as significant as we've been led to believe. We believe the relentless obsession with health is not health promoting. But it does promote profit.

Ever notice how there's a "Health and Beauty" section in big box stores like Target? These two things are commonly conflated in our culture. When people say health and fitness are important to them, what they often mean is they want to be perceived as beautiful, worthy, desirable, part of an elite group. And these things are often presented as something that can be bought. It is less about feeling good and more about being perceived as good, worthy, and financially secure. Health has, essentially, become an aesthetic.

In an April 2021 *Vanity Fair* article about how "the Silicon Valley tech rich have come to be seen almost as deities," Nick Bilton writes about the pedestaling of rich people's lifestyles and the extremes they go to in their obsession with the idea of health: "Those who push themselves to extremes—by hacking their bodies, drinking Soylent instead of consuming real food, or forgoing sustenance altogether—are not seen as odd, but considered on the bleeding edge, as if they were just doing this to show us mere mortals how in control they are of their own lives." Later in the article, Bilton shares how body hacking "first made its way into the mainstream in 1984 by way of the sci-fi subculture novel *Neuromancer* but has since leapt off the page and into Palo Alto, where everyone seems to want to outdo their cohorts by pushing their bodies to extremes. You've got the Dorseys of the world bragging about how little they eat each day, the Zuckerbergs boasting of killing their own food, and an army of nerds now wearing every tracking device imaginable—from rings that follow your sleep to real-time sugar monitoring devices you inject into your arm—and then experimenting with all forms of starvation and sleep habits to show how in control they are of their bodies. There's intermittent fasting, working under infrared heat lamps, calculating ketones, and working with "DIY surgeons" to implant magnets and microchips."[16] Tweaking health has become an extremely individualistic hobby that knows no bounds.

Does this sound like health to you? With a more critical eye on culture, it sounds obsessive, controlling, unnecessary, and violent, kind of like eating disorders, which are dangerous, life-threatening conditions. So is this really about health? And what is health anyway? If you asked a room full of doctors how they define health, there wouldn't be an easy answer. There likely wouldn't even be agreement. The answers would depend on their field of study, training curricula, identities and positionality, lived experience, world view, liberatory consciousness, and more.

To us, health is deeply personal, so we wonder, What does health mean to you? How would you define it? Assess it? What do you know—from your own lived experience—impacts your health and well-being? How has shame impacted your health? What about trauma and oppression? What has come between you and being at home in your body? What interferes with your ability to care for yourself in the ways you personally feel drawn to (as opposed to the "shoulds") that you know would make a difference in your life? There are so many institutional, societal, and structural barriers that get in the way, so be gentle as you consider these questions.

We need the medical community to reckon with the harm they've done in upholding healthism and the dominant weight paradigm, which, again, is a failed paradigm. We need the health care system to divest from diet culture so it can begin to support people in having healthier relationships with food and their bodies. A better relationship with the body promotes attuned self-care as opposed to self-neglect and self-harm. In an article titled "The Weight-Inclusive versus Weight-Normative Approach to Health," Tracy Tylka and colleagues write:

> The key is for both health care professionals and patients to appreciate the extent to which body loathing and shame is associated with reduced engagement in self-care. There is a cultural belief that people have to be dissatisfied with their weight (or any aspect of their appearance) to be motivated to improve it. This belief has not found general support in the literature; in fact, the reverse is supported: people are more likely to take care of their bodies when they appreciate and hold positive feelings toward their bodies.[17]

Self-care rooted in the dominant culture's ideals is often performative, unsustainable, and not in alignment with how our truest self wants to be cared for. When you start to think of beauty, gender, weight, health, and fitness as social constructs, it allows some space for the uprooting of these ideals. We encourage you to consider how these constructs have impacted your relationship with your body and limited the expression of your authentic self. Beginning the process of divesting from diet culture will allow a whole new world to open up.

Reading through all this might have you spinning. You might be feeling rage. You might also notice a sense of relief, as you resonate with these stories and allow a door to open within yourself. Or you may feel defensive. Maybe a combo of all of the above? We invite you to "welcome and entertain them all!" as the poet Rumi expresses in his famous poem "The Guest House," a poem about how gaining understanding of the many parts of ourselves can be likened to welcoming the many houseguests that appear at your door each day. This is your story to investigate. For now, know this: divesting is an opportunity, a time for deep reckoning, for humility, for listening, and for leaning into the discomfort of not knowing.

Before you can root into something more nourishing and affirming of your entire being, the work is to begin divesting from diet culture. From shame and perfectionism. From social constructs of gender. From constraining social discourses about beauty and desire. All these oppressive constructs have roots in white supremacy, and we cannot divest from one system of oppression without also considering how it intersects with others. In a conversation we had with Sonya Renee Taylor for our Body Trust Summit a few years back, Sonya said:

> *Fatphobia is so important because it reminds us how we are all connected to a historical system that is interrelated; as it relates to oppression that is, for the purpose of power, codifying and centralizing power and resources. And what I do when I divest from that system, personally, is I pull a small brick—a small and important brick out of the foundation of oppression. I'm part of all the hands pulling down the bricks of these systems. That, for me, is worth the work. Understanding how that personal work of de-indoctrination is part of creating the world we want to be in becomes part of that necessary motivation.*
>
> *Every time we do something counter to what these systems would have us do, we are actively engaged in this process of de-indoctrination, which is divestment. None of these systems stand up by themselves. They're not just these omniscient energies that control our lives. They are maintained by the active and passive participation of each and every one of us. We are all in one way either holding it up or tearing it down. And every time we engage in opposite action toward what that system would have us do, we're part of tearing it down. We are*

divesting from that system because the system's goal is not to nourish you. The system's goal is to nourish itself.

We are fairly certain you don't like the idea of these systems using you. And you also don't want to uphold or participate in the harm the systems create. If you are just beginning to make the connections between social justice and the dominant weight paradigm, we are glad you are here! It will take some time to unpack all of this and let it settle into your bones, especially if you've been relating to food and your body in more mainstream ways for a long time. Here are a few questions to explore:

∗ What have you gained by conforming to these social constructs? What's been lost?

∗ How has not knowing these truths "held you back and held you down"?

∗ Who benefits when you are distracted by the hustle? Who makes money off your shame?

∗ Who are you allowed to be when you realize society is the problem, not you or your body?

Here is more of Nicole K.'s body story:

I flooded my Instagram with body positive and fat role models; I unfollowed Facebook friends who talked about dieting and made fat jokes. I started to embrace the word FAT. At first I couldn't hear it without cringing. But the more I experienced people using it as a neutral descriptor of themselves versus a word that was synonymous with laziness, disgust, and hate, the more normal it felt. And then one day when I was talking to a friend, I referred to myself as fat. It just kind of slipped out and it felt powerful. Like it wasn't a word to

be feared, but a word that was embracing who I was. I was
finally speaking my truth.

When we divest, we are reconnecting to the parts of us that have been fragmented in The Hustle. We are reclaiming the elements of self that have been buried under survival and coping mechanisms and performative measures meant to protect us. We are identifying who and what in our life nourishes our sense of worthiness. We are rediscovering what lights us up and makes us feel whole again. Here are some recommendations to help you become aware of the things in your life that keep you rooted in diet culture so you can begin the process of divestment:

Reduce body checking behaviors. There are all kinds of ways people habitually monitor the body: weighing, measuring, comparing and despairing, slapping/pinching fat, trying on jeans to see if they fit, scrutinizing your body in the mirror, spending more time looking at yourself on Zoom than looking at everyone else. One of the first steps to having a more subjective experience of your body (versus an objectified experience) is to become aware of and reduce body checking behaviors.

Get rid of your scale. Or put it somewhere it is hard to access so you really, really have to think about it before you step on it. If you weigh yourself daily or weekly and stopping altogether feels too big, consider reducing the frequency and get curious about what you are really hoping you will find out by stepping on the scale. Ask yourself: Can a piece of metal and plastic that measures my relationship to gravity really tell me that I'm okay?

Unsubscribe, block, unfollow. People who are invested in diet culture receive a lot of reinforcement in their inboxes as well as from friends and the people they follow on social media. If diet-y shit shows up in your inbox, unsubscribe (and write them a note telling them why). When a friend is posting nonstop about their latest plan, unfollow for thirty days, block, or unfriend. Once you start to see just how pervasive this messaging is, you won't be able to unsee it. Over time, you can lessen your exposure to toxic posts that pull you back toward old patterns.

Curate your social media feed. Look for food- and fat-positive people to follow and fill your feed with accounts that feature a diverse array of bodies and portray all bodies in a positive light. Shoog McDaniel is a Florida-based photographer challenging the status quo by creating a stunning collection of unapologetic photos that feature transgressive bodies "being happy, enjoying their bodies, and connected to the earth." Shoog says, "The more trans, fat and queer freaks I photographed, the more I came to terms with my own identities and began to love myself."[18] Some people create a second "Body Trust" account for especially hard days when they need to safely access reinforcing messages. You can check out who we follow or head to our website for some recommendations.

Learn more about the fat acceptance movement and alternatives to diet culture. There are a lot of books and podcasts that can help you rethink what you've been taught to believe about bodies, food, weight, and health. Some of our favorites include Sonya Renee Taylor's *The Body Is Not An Apology*, Aubrey Gordon's *What We Don't Talk About When We Talk About Fat* (also check out her podcast "Maintenance Phase"), Sabrina Strings's *Fearing the Black Body*, Da'Shaun Harrison's *Belly of the Beast*, and Christy Harrison's *Anti-Diet*. You'll find more recommendations on our website, including Sirius Bonner's essay "A Brief History of the Fat Acceptance Movement."

Throw out the tools that reinforce the hustle. Delete fitness trackers, calorie counters, and weight loss apps like Noom. Recycle (or burn) diet books so nobody else has access to the harmful information in them. Stop measuring and weighing your food portions. Use measuring cups, spoons, and scales only for the purpose of cooking.

Box up clothes that do not fit. Having a closet full of clothes that don't fit sets you up for a bad (body) day and triggers thoughts about making The Plan. You may not be ready to get rid of clothes, but spending an hour or two (on a day when you are feeling resilient) going through old clothes and putting them out of sight will help prevent a shame spiral and another trip about The Cycle.

Make sure you have a few items of clothing that fit your body today. You don't have to go out and buy an entire new wardrobe, but having some clothes that fit your "today body" can make a big difference in how you feel about yourself. Button and bra extenders can help make some clothes fit more comfortably now too. You deserve to feel comfortable as you do your daily activities.

Remove yourself from conversations centered around weight and perfecting food/bodies. You may have to take a break from spending time with certain people in your life while you are newer to this work and you're not yet fully vested. What you are learning here is countercultural, and when the seeds are just beginning to take root, you will benefit from some protection. You may not be able to fully disengage from every conversation happening around you, but reducing your exposure over time will do wonders for your mental health.

Challenge your gender training. Exploring how gender norms have limited your ability to fully express yourself and participate in life is part of the reclamation process. Here are some questions for you to consider: What are some of the subtle and overt messages you received about gender roles and rules growing up? What memories do you have around expectations to behave a certain way based on your gender? What happened to you, or the people around you, when someone didn't conform to gender expectations? What gender differences did you observe in terms of food and eating behaviors, permission for pleasure, etc.?

Practice body gratitude. Changing the way you feel about your body is going to take some time. Something more immediately accessible is to start to notice the amazing ways your body shows up for you every day. Start a little body gratitude practice. At the end of the day, reflect on and acknowledge one or two things your body did to support you. This will help you move toward a more layered understanding of your body and open the door for more neutral or positive experiences over time.

Stretch the edges of your body positivity until all bodies are included and affirmed. We all have work to do to make this world more inclusive and equitable, including learning how internalized dominance and anti-fat bias live in and work through us. When you find yourself reacting in habitually negative ways to your own body and other people's bodies, name the objectification and dehumanization happening ("I see you, fatphobia"). Instead of judging yourself for it, remember you've been harmed by these systems too and are healing. With curiosity, ask yourself: Who benefits when I view myself and others in this way? What do I get when I think and believe this? What do I lose? And keep finding ways to expose yourself to images that challenge the status quo.

We wouldn't expect you to do all the things on this list immediately. Pick two or three of the recommendations you feel most drawn to right now (maybe not the hardest ones) to experiment with this week. You can return to this list in the future to get more ideas as you feel ready.

We thought it might be helpful to hear from Savala Nolan, author of *Don't Let It Get You Down,* who has worked with Body Trust concepts for six years and speaks to retreat participants about the journey of liberating herself from diet culture. She was put on her first diet at four years of age.

I began [this work] very slowly and through fits and starts, sometimes with anxiety and sometimes with joy, sometimes with fear and sometimes with ecstasy, like, "Oh my God, my body can just exist. I don't have to fix it. I can have ice cream as often as I want. I can be fat." Realizing my fear of fatness was related to my internalized fear of Blackness created a big shift for me. I'm Black and I'm mixed, but I identify as Black. Making the connection between the fatphobia I have lived with my whole life and the anti-Black racism I have been steeped in and swallowing enabled me to find a political handhold on my own liberation that I couldn't quite grasp when it was just about fatphobia. Somehow it also being about racism made me go, okay, I'm really done. Although "done," you know, is a process—but it gave me extra fire once I figured that out.

I went through a period of intense anger for how I'd been lied to, both within my family and just from living in this culture. This reckoning with the lies has been complicated, not clean and tidy. For instance, I was angry that I was turned into a chronic dieter because one of the outcomes of chronic dieting tends to be weight gain. So, like, if I had not gone on so many diets, what would I weigh now? Would I still be fat? Then at some point I realized, oh wait, I'm still hung up on the "fat is bad" thing, so I had to unpack that.

After anger, I felt grief. I began to reckon with the impact all of these lies had on my own life. I began very, very, very slowly to actually shed fatphobia. That is 110 percent still a process. But I went from being someone who would burst into tears if a doctor told me that I could stand to lose ten pounds to being someone who just describes themselves as fat, neutrally. This is a massive shift after thirty-plus years of being unable to bear someone insinuating that I was fat or using that word to describe me.

When I was new to this work, with my feet freshly planted in new terrain, any wind in the atmosphere (diet talk, fatphobia) would knock me around quite intensely. Over time, though, I've become harder to knock around. I changed my media consumption, who I follow on Instagram, who I'm close to, who I'm willing to talk about the journey with. I have people in my life that I am not quite as close to as I used to be because of their deep involvement with diet culture. With all of that stuff and with time—the more days and weeks and months and years I've spent doing this work—my roots have gotten so much deeper and they are in this much healthier soil. So when a huge gust of wind comes, it doesn't rock me anymore. If somebody called me fat now as an insult, it just doesn't impact me, whereas before it would crush me. The culture is always trying to pull me out of the soil of liberation. The work is hard, but the longer you are in the journey and the deeper your roots get, the easier it is to just not feel like you're in a hurricane when the diet culture stuff is all around you.

This process of reclaiming my body, of no longer thinking of myself as a public park that has to look pretty for everyone to walk by and see, has been like the color coming on in my life when my world was previously black and white (you know, like in the movies). This has been like the lights coming on in my life. And as hard as it can be to be fat, I would never go back to my dieting days, never, ever, ever, never, ever, ever. And I did not see that coming.

I have so much more space for creativity. I'm 100 percent sure I would not have written a book if I was still dieting. I have more space for political engagement with the world. So the process, while difficult and complex, has been really, really rich, and really beautiful.

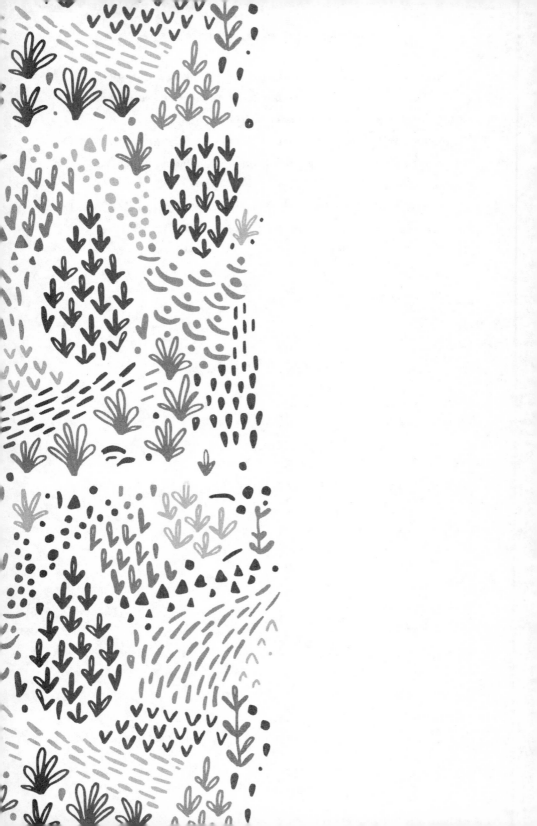

CHAPTER 5

Reckoning with Your Eating

and I said to my body. softly. "I want to be your friend."
it took a long breath. and replied, "I have been
waiting my whole life for this."

—NAYYIRAH WAHEED

T
ake a moment to think about a few of your favorite eating experiences (maybe before food got so damn complicated) and notice all the details of the experience. Where were you? Who were you with? What was the atmosphere like? What did you have to eat and drink? What else can you remember that made the meal particularly special?

Chances are that your favorite meals are ones where the atmosphere in which you were eating was just as nourishing as the food itself. You might remember the loved ones you were eating with or the sense of being cared for, the stimulating conversation, the laughter and tears, the view from the table, the sun setting as you ate, the band playing in the background, the attentive service, perfect weather, and more. French gourmet Jean-Anthelme Brillat-Savarin said, in essence,

"Animals feed while humans dine." We come together and commune through food. The table is where connections are made, where deep conversations happen and minds are expanded or changed. It is where we share our sorrows and our joy. Every culture has customs and rites that center around food. It can often be the very thing that defines us as a people.

M. F. K. Fisher writes, "It seems to me that our three basic needs, for food and security and love, are so mixed and mingled and intertwined that we cannot straightly think of one without the others. So it happens that when I write about hunger, I am really writing about love and the hunger for it . . . and then the warmth and richness and fine reality of hunger satisfied . . . There is a communion of more than our bodies when bread is broken and wine drunk."[1]

There's a scene toward the end of the animated film *Ratatouille*, when the curmudgeonly food critic, Anton Ego, known for giving only bad restaurant reviews, is served a main course of ratatouille. At first he is perplexed at the chef's choice. But when he takes his first bite, he flashes back to a memory of himself as a young boy coming home with a banged-up knee from a bicycle accident, tears in his eyes and clearly shaken up. He sits down at the kitchen table and his mom brings him a comforting bowl of ratatouille. The scene returns to him in the restaurant, where he drops his pen in astonishment, his eyes filled with tears. He smiles, dives back into the dish with childlike wonder, and eats the rest with the most delightful look on his face.

When we dumb food down and reduce it to the sum of its ingredients or nutritional components, we miss out on so much. We miss the intense connections between food and culture and the layers of nourishment food and eating offer. We miss out on the traditions that center around food. Eating is not—and should never be—just about survival. For human beings, food is flavored with complex meaning. It tells the story of your ancestors, your culture, your history. The bottom line: When people mess with your food, they are messing with your life in ways rarely anticipated or understood. In a speech about culinary justice, African American culinary historian Michael Twitty said,

> Our food was a way that our ancestors preserved themselves. They took our names, they took our religion, they took our gods, but they didn't take our food . . . Food connects us. Food liberates us. And by sharing our pasties and our collard greens . . . by sharing our food traditions and talking about where we've come from and where we are going, we remind ourselves that we are one family with one destiny and one aim.[2]

When Black people are diagnosed with a health condition that prompts a referral to a dietitian, they are often presented with a Eurocentric view of a healthy diet. In her course Culture, Equity, Diversity, and Race in Dietetics, Rosie Mensah shared her sixty-year-old father's experience seeing a white Canadian dietitian about a low-sodium diet after being diagnosed with high blood pressure. After sharing what he typically eats in a day, he was told to stop eating fufu—a traditional dish from his homeland Ghana made with plantain or cassava—and to eat brown rice instead because "it is better for him." The dietitian neglected to do any research to understand how the dish was prepared and see how one might reduce the sodium in it. Instead, they suggested he give up a traditional food that connects him to his culture, his people. He left feeling frustrated, misunderstood, and judged, and never returned for a follow-up visit.

The training most dietitians and nutritional professionals receive is steeped in classism and white supremacy and fails to acknowledge the complexity of people's lives and what support will truly serve them. Society tends to minimize the power of food, and many want to reduce it to simply fuel when it is so much more. One client we worked with years ago complained of having "a thing with ice cream." Because of some health concerns, she believed that eating a bowl of ice cream every night was not a good idea. She tried to sometimes skip it and said, "Every night that bowl of ice cream calls to me." In addition to talking about how when we think or are told we can't have something our desire for it increases, we asked about her relationship with ice cream throughout her life. She gasped and said, "I totally forgot this, but ice cream was one of the only things my dad could eat in his last weeks of life before he died of cancer. Every night we would enjoy a bowl of ice cream together, and I think after he passed, ice cream became my way of staying connected to him."

In society's narrow definition of "healthy eating," this behavior is pathologized instead of seen as a normal human experience. We all eat for emotional reasons. We celebrate the promotion by going out for a nice dinner. There are elaborate feasts at weddings. People eat food together to grieve the loss of a loved one, sharing stories that bring laughter, tears, and healing. Food is something human beings turn toward or away from to soothe, comfort, or numb ourselves. This form of coping to meet our emotional needs can go as far back as before we were verbal.

Each and every living person has a relationship with food and eating. Nobody gets out of this relationship, no matter how hard they might try. Just after we are born, one of the first ways we connect and communicate with another human is through nourishment. How attuned your caregivers were, whether or not they ate with you, what they modeled at the table, and what the environment was like when eating together set a foundation for what your relationship with food and eating would be like as an adult.

If you've experienced food insecurity or childhood food neglect, research shows there's an increased risk of all types of eating disorders. Sometimes families have sufficient resources for food, but the way they managed food in the household mimicked food insecurity—they didn't provide enough food consistently and predictably and kids couldn't anticipate when they would be eating next. Maybe because the parents were working multiple jobs to make ends meet. Or life was busy or chaotic. Other times it is because the caregivers have their own disrupted relationship with food and/or they were anxious about your growth pattern, weight, or health. Regardless of the reason, the resulting inconsistent and restrained feeding practices can have lasting impacts.

Combine all this with living in a world steeped in anti-fatness and diet culture and it is a recipe for a fraught relationship with food and eating. Few of us are immune. There's a lot to unpack as you reckon with your relationship with food and reclaim your identity as an eater. It wouldn't surprise us if the idea of exploring this more deeply brings up fear, shame, or confusion.

We wonder, What words would you use to describe your current relationship with food and eating? What does it feel like right now? When we ask this question in our Body Trust groups, people say things like insecure, insufficient, scared, hopeless, baffled, unsettled, anxious, exhausting, impatient, disconnected, judgmental, and trapped.

How do you want this relationship to feel? Most often we hear things like relaxed, content, obsession-free, accepting, confident, nonjudgmental, grateful, open-minded, authentic, connected, and joyful.

Many of the people we work with spend the bulk of their time obsessing over their choices, preoccupied with getting it right. Their shelves are filled with every nutrition/diet book on the market while their pantries are mostly empty. They receive dozens of emails each week with diet and nutrition tips, while their refrigerators hold only a few of the most basic items. Some weeks they are vegan, other weeks they are doing paleo or keto. Some days they decide gluten free is the way to be, and then when that gets old, it is sugar and dairy that need to be avoided. And between each diet-of-the-moment, they rarely return to the flexibility of normal eating. They swing from rigidity and perfectionism to an attitude of whatever or fuck it, and then back to rigidity and perfectionism.

For some, the obsession with eating correctly gets so extreme they track the quality of their stools (yes, there are poop trackers) and make adjustments to their diet in the hopes of producing the perfect poop.

Food rules become more and more extreme. The list of foods they are willing to eat becomes quite limited. Physician Steven Bratman coined the term "orthorexia nervosa" to describe "a pathological fixation on eating proper food" when his eating behaviors became so extreme he wouldn't eat any vegetable that had been out of his garden for more than fifteen minutes. Because our society puts people hustling for health on a pedestal and deems them morally superior with their "clean" lifestyles, the disordered aspects of these behaviors are difficult for most to see. Bratman says, "Many of the most unbalanced people I have ever met are those who have devoted themselves to healthy eating."[3]

Other clients navigate the world unaware of and/or ignoring their food needs, not really thinking about it, winging it from meal to meal, pushing their body to extremes, attempting for as long as possible to be immune to their body's requirement for food until their body just can't take it anymore. If your early childhood experiences included abuse and neglect, or you have a history of food insecurity, you may not know how to meet your needs, how to feed yourself regularly, and perhaps believe it is better not to need anything or anyone.

Body Trust is repair work focused on healing your relationship with food and your body rather than perfecting it. We are repairing the damage done living in a culture that doesn't trust your body, that disrupts your ability to feel at home in your body, that undermines your agency and feels threatened by body sovereignty—the freedom to do what you want with your body. To love who you want. Eat what you want. Move your body if you want to, in the ways you want to. Wear what you want. Have sex when and with whomever you want. Unapologetically. This is your body. It is where *you* live. It is you.

Over the span of your lifetime, you've probably been inundated with all kinds of nutrition tips, health advice, and strategies to lose weight for good. We didn't write this book to help you perform health by improving what you are eating. We are not interested in helping you acquiesce to the culture. We do not believe it is possible to repair your relationship with food and your body by using a plan to make it into what the dominant culture thinks it should be. We are pretty sure that would just send you on another trip around The Cycle. What this book will do is reconnect you to your own knowing, your deepest truths, and your inner wisdom so you can find a personal food, health, and wellness philosophy that is flexible enough to work for you . . . in your unique life. A sustainable philosophy centered on pleasure and nourishment, not deprivation and restraint. Regardless of what you've been through in your life and what food and eating is like for you today, we promise it can get better. This chapter will help you reckon with the dieting mind and your food caretaking behaviors. We will talk about why it is important to give yourself unconditional permission to eat and enjoy food. We challenge the food addiction model and wrap up with some recommendations for navigating the world of food and eating so you can figure out what works best for you moving forward.

Reckoning with the Dieting Mind

Our attitudes, practices, and rituals around food are a window into our most basic beliefs about the world and ourselves. Many of us were indoctrinated into diet culture before we were old enough to give informed consent. Regardless of your personal history with dieting and disordered eating, growing up in diet culture gives rise to a dieting mind: thinking about food and eating in binary ways like good or bad, right or wrong, making choices based primarily on calories/fat/points/macros or red/yellow/green categories, etc., experiencing guilt and shame after eating, focusing on how you will make up for your "bad" choices, and wondering if you deserve or have earned the right to eat. It can show up as tracking your food, calories, etc., or white-knuckling to restrain yourself during a meal when you are still hungry or wanting more because it tastes so damn good. The more we engage with food in this way, the more deeply ingrained this mentality is.

Many of the "this isn't a diet, it's a lifestyle" programs out there today co-opt anti-diet language while continuing to collude with the dieting mind, and this includes the medical community and weight loss researchers. Psychologist Deb Burgard, one of the founders of the Health at Every Size movement, says, "We prescribe for fat bodies what we diagnose as an eating disorder in thin bodies."

We tell fat people to weigh themselves daily and thin people with eating disorders to stop weighing obsessively.

We tell fat people to track their food and calories every day while telling smaller-bodied people with eating disorders to stop doing this.

We tell people to chew gum or drink some tea or water when they are hungry while discouraging thin people with eating disorders from doing these things to numb hunger and avoid eating.

We tell fat people to basically develop a compulsive exercise disorder while imposing exercise restrictions on smaller-bodied people with eating disorders.

The TV show *The Biggest Loser* is a prime example of how the culture upholds eating disordered behavior in the name of weight loss. Contestants on the show severely restrict their food while exercising at compulsive levels. It is considered entertainment by some, and inspiration for others, to watch fat people vomit or pass out from the extremes they put their bodies through in the name of health via weight loss. THIS. IS. NOT. HEALTH. This is what eating disorders look like, and eating disorders are life-threatening conditions. Regardless of whether your new plan is called a diet, any program that promotes and promises weight loss is a diet, and as such, it will keep you rooted in the dieting mind. As we shared in the last chapter, Noom is the latest program that many people think is different because they've brilliantly marketed the "psychology behind it." But folks who have tried Noom tell us they are encouraged to weigh themselves daily as well as track their food. Same shit, different program. We predict their data will be no different, and with time, show that people do not maintain any weight lost two to five years later.

Take a moment to think about all the things you've tried to perfect your body, your food, and your eating habits. If helpful, write them all down on a piece of paper and then reflect on these questions: How different or similar were these programs and plans? How long were you able to sustain them? What did you like about them? What didn't you like about them? What would eventually get in the way of you pulling it off in the long run? Who do you blame when you can't pull it off?

Restrictive eating plans are not sustainable for most people. There's a honeymoon phase and then we tire of them. We get tired of having to keep certain foods off-limits. We get tired of tracking our food, being hungry, eating the same thing every day because it is easier to know how it adds up. We get tired of always having to plan our food and skip out on social activities to "stay on track." And our body tires of this too. In an attempt to survive famine, the body eventually kicks in with metabolic adaptations that prevent further weight loss, even if you white-knuckle through the discomfort and sustain the changes in your eating pattern. When we hit "the plateau," we are even more likely to abandon ship (weight maintenance isn't as thrilling as losing weight) and swing back over to the "fuck it" plan. With our metabolism slowed, any weight that was lost comes back on . . . plus more. Then it's rinse and repeat.

And every time we repeat this pattern, there are negative impacts. "A large body of literature has connected weight cycling directly to compromised health, including higher mortality, higher risk of osteoporotic fractures and gallstone attacks, loss of muscle tissue, hypertension, chronic inflammation, and some forms of cancer. . . . Weight cycling also has been shown to be connected to compromised physical health and psychological well-being. . . . Weight loss led to reductions in metabolic energy expenditure . . . mak[ing] it difficult for their participants to maintain their newly suppressed weight."[4]

Food deprivation not only injures our health and our metabolism, it also significantly harms our psychological well-being and our relationship with food and eating in ways that are long lasting. The Minnesota

Starvation Experiment by researcher Ancel Keys during World War II was designed to show the impacts of famine on the human body. Thirty-two white men of "sound mind and body" who were "conscientious objectors to the war" volunteered to be observed during a six-month period of semi-starvation. The study began with three months where the participants were allowed to eat their typical quantities and whatever foods they wanted, and then their calories were cut in half for six months. The men reported intense food cravings and obsessive thoughts about food. They were even collecting recipes. Most men in the 1940s probably didn't look at recipes, let alone collect them!

During the six months of semi-starvation, the men developed bizarre eating patterns, like pushing food around the plate to make it last longer or ravenously gulping their food. Their personalities changed; they were moody, anxious, irritable. Some had a flat affect. They lost interest in sex. And their metabolic rates decreased by 40 percent. When food was liberated and they were allowed to eat at will, they reported an insatiable hunger and the fear that food would not be available. Many found it hard to stop eating. It took the majority of them five months for their eating to normalize, and some never returned to baseline.

Now just think of this: after one six-month period of food restriction (which, by the way, the caloric level was what modern weight loss diets recommend for men today), it took them close to half a year to normalize their eating. One six-month period of food deprivation took equally as long to recover from. What we've noticed is that the people who cut their calories to lose weight rarely return to normal eating after bottoming out, especially after multiple previous attempts. There's usually the backlash period of eating, including "the last supper" before the next plan begins. All of this is to say that if your food has been restricted and restrained for long periods of time throughout your life, we strongly encourage you to allow time for you and your body to recover. We understand the desire for a shortcut, but it has taken a while to get here. It's gonna take some time for things to root in and settle.

In order to have a different relationship with food, you must reckon with and divest from the diet mentality. This means that the work right now is to continually set your thoughts about weight and health to the side (tell yourself "not now") so you can start to connect with and listen to your own knowing and inner wisdom. Get curious about how you decide when, what, and how much to eat. Start asking yourself if you like what you are eating. Notice how often you walk away from a meal feeling full but not at all satisfied. How often do you "suck it up" and eat things you do not enjoy in the name of health or weight loss? In the long run, giving up pleasure in the name of weight loss/health is not sustainable for most. For now, when you notice these old diet-y thoughts, say, "Oh, hello, dieting mind, I see you" or "Nope, we are not doing that right now."

We want you to have a chance to get to know who you are and what your eating is like without all the noise. When you turn toward your body and listen for input and feedback about when you need to eat, what you want, how much you need to feel satisfied, and how different foods make you feel, you can make choices in an embodied, connected way. Take it one meal and one day at a time. Try to approach each eating opportunity with a blank slate and see it as a new opportunity to practice awareness, connection, and choice. Then notice what happens. Stay curious. Over time, you'll have more experiences and more practice, and it is through these small, consistent acts that you'll rebuild trust between you and your body.

Reckoning with Food Caretaking

We wouldn't be surprised if, when you hear the phrase "food caretaking," you roll your eyes, immediately feel exhausted, or think of those days when you spent hours meticulously planning and preparing your meals for the week. When we use the phrase "food caretaking," we are talking about the things you do to make sure food is available and that you'll get enough to eat throughout the day. This doesn't mean obsessively planning out your food for the day, week, or month. It doesn't mean reporting your plan to your sponsor and clearing any changes you want to make before you eat. What it does mean is having some idea of how you are going to meet your needs for nourishment throughout the day.

Many of the people we work with have such a complicated history with food and eating that when they leave the house for long periods of time, whether it's to go to work or run errands, there isn't any acknowledgment that at some point they will get hungry and need to eat. We see parents packing their kid's lunch and snacks without even considering making and bringing something for themselves. Mixed in there is the mindset that *less is better* or *it's better not to eat* and so eating is put off for as long as possible. They wait and wait and push their bodies up to the point where they just can't take it anymore. And it is from this place that they are faced with decisions about what to eat.

This kind of food caretaking mimics food insecurity. So while food may be available, or you have money to purchase food, your body does not know this. It thinks there must be a famine—that you are unable to access food—and when food finally becomes available, it can be hard not to eat really fast, eat past full, and be left feeling stuffed and uncomfortable.

Caring for our food needs can feel like a full-time job in an already busy and overwhelming life. Combine this with living in a culture that changes its opinion every few years (if not months) on what is the healthiest way to eat, and food becomes even more confusing and challenging to get on the table. It's no wonder so many of us throw our hands up in the air and say fuck it. Ellyn Satter gets straight to the point when she says, "When the joy goes out of eating, nutrition suffers."[5]

Over time, food trends and fad diets contradict each other and people are left with so much conflicting information that it can be hard to know what's right and what's nonsense. In the 1990s, carbs were okay and we were supposed to eat low-fat. We had things like SnackWells and olestra. Then in early 2000, it became all about eating low-carb. The Atkins Diet made a comeback (it debuted in the 1970s). Then we had South Beach. More recently, people are all about eating paleo or going keto. Gluten was the demon for a while, and the gluten-free fad benefited people with celiac disease who've been desperate for good tasting, gluten-free substitutes, but had many others unnecessarily eliminating an entire food group in the name of health.

We hear sugar is addictive, that it lights up the same part of the brain as heroin! (Listening to good music, getting a hug, and winning a prize also light up this part of the brain! More on this later.) The people who eat a raw food diet think those who are macrobiotic are ill-informed, and vice versa. Dana worked at what was then called a "health food store" in the early nineties. One customer wanted the carrots cut an inch from the top because "the tops were poison," and the next customer wanted the whole carrot including the greens to be juiced because "there were so many wonderful nutrients that we miss out on when we throw the tops away." So many contradicting opinions!

The more people engage in fad diets and food trends, the more they talk about it, and one reason for this is because food deprivation increases preoccupation with food. There's also a moral superiority some folks have about their eating—it puffs up people's sense of self. We've got people with large followings talking about keto and intermittent fasting, "What I Eat in a Day" videos, Whole30, Macros, or whatever the fuck the diet-of-the-day is at the time you are reading this book. The idea being that food control is synonymous with excellence, discipline, and eliteness.

Dinner parties have become impossible to host in some communities because everyone has something they avoid eating and all these different food philosophies and preferences compete with one another, making cooking an exhaustive nightmare. Parents are telling their kids they have allergies so they don't eat the foods they think are bad for them.

(There's no such thing as a sugar allergy.) We live in the land of or-thorexia (Pacific Northwest) and Hilary's son came home from school asking why he was the only kid in his class without a food allergy. He actually had some FOMO about this!

We'd be remiss if we didn't call out the class differences in these ex-periences. Not everyone has the time, energy, or money to spend plan-ning, purchasing, and preparing their food when they are working two to three jobs to pay the bills, helping their kids with various school proj-ects and activities, dealing with environmental racism, and attending to the needs of their community. Financial privilege brings with it the time and resources to obsess about perfecting food and living a healthy lifestyle. Gwyneth Paltrow attempted to eat on $29 a week, which is the amount SNAP participants try to survive on, and lasted four days.[6]

Human beings have a knack for making things harder than they need to be, and it is astounding to observe how people will take di-etary advice from anyone who is willing to dish it out, regardless of their background or qualifications. The majority of helping profession-als and teachers have little to no nutrition education. One study, pub-lished in The Lancet, stated that "nutrition is insufficiently incorporated into medical education."[7] But because everybody eats, everybody has an opinion about the right way to eat. What gets spouted off as nutrition advice today is more personal philosophy than solid science with a body of evidence supporting it. Nutrition is actually a relatively young science and there's still so much we do not know.

We are not saying that nutrition doesn't have some impact on our health and well-being. But there is no one right way to eat for every-body. What makes one person feel their best may make another person lethargic and foggy headed. Eating is deeply personal. This is your re-lationship with food. We will not be giving any dietary advice in this chapter because it will just be more noise right now. And we trust you to figure out what works best for you, especially once you've given yourself a chance to do some of this healing work. What we want to offer here are some suggestions to help you explore food and eating, and better care for your food needs.

Increase Access to Food

Food deprivation isn't always related to diet culture, the pursuit of thinness, or the desire to feel in control. Sometimes the lack of adequate intake was due to our caregivers not having enough money and resources to give us consistent, stable access to food. Some of you may still struggle financially to meet all your needs and find yourself stretching food to make it last, prioritizing your children's food needs over your own, eating the same thing several days in a row because that's all you have, or needing to use the little money you have to pay for bills and non-food expenses.

Carolyn Becker Black, PhD, and Keesha Middlemass, PhD, are researchers working with the San Antonio Food Bank, shining a light on the connections between food insecurity and eating disorders. They have found that people who experience food insecurity have an increased risk of any type of eating disorder and higher levels of binge eating disorder. Cycles of scarcity and abundance likely contribute to this risk.[8]

Research has also shown that childhood food neglect is associated with a higher risk of an eating disorder later in life than those without a history of food neglect. If there was not enough food, or if your parents and caregivers were not attuned to your needs, or they left you for long periods of time to fend for yourself because they were working multiple jobs to keep you housed, you may have never learned how to meet your needs. Or you may have come from households with enough money and resources for food but your parents and caregivers did not consistently provide enough nourishment to meet your needs. They may have had chaotic feeding patterns themselves and they were just feeding you in the best way they could. They may have denied you snacks or seconds or desserts because they were concerned about your growth or weight, and while there was enough food available, you were not allowed to meet your needs. Child feeding expert Ellyn Satter has found that when parents' feeding practices mimic food insecurity, the child is more likely to struggle with regulating their eating. When kids have access to regular meals and snacks, they know what to expect every day. They eat according to their hunger level and food preferences and are more likely to grow up to have good relationships with food: "positive, comfortable, and flexible with eating as well as matter-of-fact and reliable about getting enough to eat of enjoyable food."[9]

Our early childhood experiences have a huge impact on what our relationship with food and eating will be like for us as adults. Artist, writer, dissonant doula, and agitator of healthism Isabel Abbott writes:

> i was raised in extreme poverty, as well as an environment of profound abuse and neglect, and i have very clear memories of being hungry, of going hungry, of there not being food to eat, of looking for food in other people's trash, of never having what was needed, while being assaulted with so much of what i did not want and could not fight off.
>
> this created a completely distorted relationship with my own body, with food, with experiences of safety in my own body. i would never have been able to tell you when i was hungry or what i was hungry for. i devoured food and yet didn't know it as something required to live. by the time i was twenty, i began hoarding food in my apartment, unable to ever trust there would be more.
>
> learning to eat was how i learned to live.
>
> and it has been a long and disjointed experience, that took so many years to heal. mostly, to learn that i was allowed food, that i would be able to provide food for myself, and that i could eat what i wanted when i wanted and believe there would be more later. in this way, to tend to my relationship with food and my own body was to mend my relationship with self, to grow trust. this is what healing was for me.[10]

Our first priority in healing your relationship with food is making sure you have access to enough food so you can eat regularly throughout the day. Giving your body the consistent message that food is available reduces food preoccupation and deprivation-based eating. This means purchasing foods you enjoy, not just the ones you, your friends and family, or society at large think you should be eating. If your ideas about what you should be eating make it harder for you to get food on the table and feed yourself regularly, take it as a sign that it's not working for you. Lay it down for now so you can focus on getting enough food to meet your needs. Work to divest from ideas and beliefs that get in the way of you feeding yourself regularly: less is better, carbs are bad, I should only eat fresh food, etc. You'd be surprised how this alone can change your attitude toward food caretaking, reduce some of the resistance to making meals, and open the door for more possibilities.

If it is possible, go to the grocery store regularly (once a week) to ensure you have enough food in your home to give you some variety and choices for meals and snacks. Doing a little planning and making lists (more on this later) will help you access meals that appeal to you and make the grocery store less overwhelming. If you are looking to lower food bills, buy store brands, use rewards cards and coupons, compare brands by the unit prices (usually on the shelf tag). If you have space to store and use food before it spoils, buy in bulk or purchase larger quantities when things you use/eat often are on sale. Shop seasonally and locally. And to reduce spoilage, check expiration dates before purchasing (grab from the back!).

If you don't want to have to think about what you are going to eat every time you get hungry, you can increase your access to food by creating a food bag (a concept we learned from Jane Hirschmann, Carol Munter, and Karin Kratina). What's a food bag? It is a bag of food that you curate with some of your favorite things to eat and carry with you throughout the day. Be sure to include a variety of flavors, textures, and amounts. Your bag could have cookies, nuts, fresh fruit, trail mix, pretzels, chips, cut-up veggies, string cheese, yogurt, nut butter, cheese puffs, fruit leather, crackers, chocolate, beef jerky, granola bars, and more. Make sure you have foods that are sweet and others that are savory, as well as a variety of textures (crunchy, chewy, and creamy). That way, when you get hungry, you can look in the bag, notice what draws your attention, and eat what sounds good to you in the moment. A food bag doesn't just ensure you have consistent access to food, but that you also have choices. Sometimes you'll want something sweet and chewy, and other times you'll be in the mood for salty and crunchy. Sometimes one item from the bag will be enough. Other times, you'll need several things to feel satisfied. Having a variety of items in your bag will help you feel less deprived and you'll also get to connect with your appetite and experiment with different choices.

When you start getting enough to eat on a regular basis, you'll feel less preoccupied with food, which frees up time and energy to focus on things you are passionate about and really matter to you. The bottom line: fed is best.

Unconditional Permission to Eat and Enjoy Food

One way to increase access to food is to give yourself unconditional permission to eat and enjoy food.[11] All human beings have a right to access enough enjoyable food to meet their needs without experiencing guilt or shame. We appreciate how the Toronto-based organization Food-Share talks about this in their statement about food justice: "Body positive food justice means greater access to food choices without shame! It means removing systemic barriers to having greater food options, without telling people what they should or should not eat."[12]

When people begin to explore Body Trust, many believe they already give themselves permission to eat what they want, but when we investigate further, it doesn't quite match our version. When one client was new to this concept, she was craving cupcakes and decided to stop by a store on the way home. After she walked up to the counter to take in all the options, she wanted to try three flavors. But then a wave of shame passed over her when she realized that if she bought only three, the person boxing up her cupcakes would know they were just for her. So she ordered a dozen cupcakes to make it look like she was taking them to a birthday party. Another client loved this chocolate nut bar from a local bakery. But the sweet treat was mostly off-limits. They allowed themselves to eat it once a week if, and only if, they met their lofty running goals.

This isn't the form of permission we are advocating for here, where you have to meet certain conditions to eat, or you have rules about how often or how much you eat (this is the dieting mind at play). When you've done the work to neutralize food and truly have unconditional permission to eat and enjoy it, you eat what you want without conditions of how much and how often. You don't put up false food fronts, where you deny yourself the foods you want and perform healthy eating when you are dining with others, only to go home and binge on the food you really wanted. And your eating experiences are free of guilt or shame—before, during, and after eating. You show up with a blank slate to each eating episode. There's no making up for the past and there are no last suppers because the next diet isn't starting tomorrow.

For many, giving yourself unconditional permission to eat is the scariest part of the work, because when you start to ask yourself what sounds good, you are going to want all the things you've not been allowed to have. You are healing from years of deprivation. It's going to take some time for eating to feel calm and settled. Remember, you can't read about this stuff and embody it. It takes practice. And if you let yourself experiment with the concept of unconditional permission to eat, the experiences, collected over time, will help you rebuild trust and be more connected to *your* yeses, noes, and not nows.

A Word about Food Addiction

If you've struggled with food and eating for a long time, you've likely found yourself thinking you have a food addiction. And we believe you when you say you feel addicted to food. This is certainly the way main-stream society frames a person's inability to "control" their eating. We have medical professionals, 12-step programs, so-called health and life-style gurus, and highly reputable academic institutions using the addiction model to talk about how people relate to food. It has become fairly common for people to say certain foods are "addictive" in casual conversation. This gets reinforced in food commercials that warn consumers how hard it is to stop eating their products once you start. So many mouthpieces in our world are absolutely certain that we will all be out of control with food if we do not practice restraint and control. So it is no wonder that many of us end up believing that food can be overpowering and dangerous to our systems. This reinforces unnecessary vigilance, which is ultimately not supportive to your health and well-being.

It is true that human beings turn toward food for comfort, soothing, or to check out sometimes. Eating can land us back in our bodies and be grounding. Sometimes food is simply where comfort is available. Food can signal a break and may be the only time you get a moment to yourself to pause and breathe and just be. When you are trying to expand your coping strategies beyond food, sometimes saying, "I'm doing this now because I need to do something" is enough to reduce shame and prevent another trip around The Cycle. Eating in response to emotions should not be pathologized, but accepted as human. And note: the eating that happens in response to food deprivation—trying to be "good" all day and not getting enough to eat—is not emotional eating. It is simply eating.

The truth is, dietary restraint and food restriction are surefire ways to "feel addicted to food." Eating disorder experts know restrictive and restrained eating leads to food preoccupation, eating in secrecy, and lots of guilt and shame, which triggers plans for not doing it again. Then the "last supper" eating ensues and this just adds to the mounting evidence that we can't be trusted and need a plan for abstinence. The Merriam-Webster dictionary defines "abstain" as "to refrain deliberately and often with an effort of self-denial from an action or practice." But how does one abstain from food when we are biologically wired to eat and meet our needs? It is actually a sign of health when we can't pull it off. The fact that food is rewarding is our body's way of ensuring we're motivated enough to seek out the nourishment and fuel we need in order to stay alive! Allowing for, and even prioritizing, pleasurable eating that is attuned to our bodies' signals encourages a long-term, balanced relationship with food that allows for consistent, flexible nourishment without rigidity and restriction.

The few studies endorsing the "food addiction treatment model" have not considered and controlled for peoples' history with food, chronic dieting behaviors, and disordered eating. Binge eating disorder (BED) is *not* an impulse control disorder, even though some researchers and eating disorder treatment centers want to frame it as such. Most eating disorder professionals know that the most effective way to treat any eating disorder, including BED, is by *reducing* restriction and dietary restraint, allowing for more flexible eating, and reincorporating once "off-limits" foods back into regular eating patterns.

Despite popular rhetoric, the way out of this predictable pattern is not to pull the reins tighter, which is what most 12-step programs centered around the concept of food addiction and compulsive eating recommend. The recommendation for more monitoring, more control, more rigidity, and stricter rules is harmful collusion with the dieting mind.

When Stacey arrived in Dana's office, she was desperate for something different. She'd tried everything to get her eating under control, including two weight loss surgeries. She'd long attended 12-step programs for "compulsive overeaters" and had multiple sponsors drop her for not following their rules, like clearing any last-minute changes to her meal plan with them before eating. When Stacey wanted mustard on her sandwich instead of mayo, she had to get her sponsor's approval. When she first heard about the concept of unconditional permission to eat and enjoy food, she thought there was no way it would work for her.

She wanted control so badly, and she desperately wanted to lose weight. But she also knew she was done with the status quo. That she couldn't keep doing what she'd been doing for twenty-plus years and expect it to suddenly start working for her. So while she was hesitant, she dove in with both feet. We worked to increase access to food, and she started to eat regular meals and snacks. Her hunger and fullness cues came back online. She was giving herself unconditional permission to eat and enjoy food. She ate more foods that sounded good (versus what she thought she should eat). And she was frustrated that she couldn't seem to pass up any free food in the lunchroom, even when she didn't like it. We'd review the concept of C- work and encourage her to resist the urge to make a plan. That the only plan was to listen and to keep reminding her body that she was done with deprivation. That from now on, she was allowed to eat what she wanted when she wanted it, so it was okay to say *no* or *not now* to food. One day, after a few months of experimenting with different choices, Stacey came in and said, "Tonight's headline news: Stacey left food alone in the lunchroom." She did this not because she was "being good" but because it was a connected choice, rooted in sovereignty, not deprivation. This had felt impossible before she'd done the foundational work of giving herself unconditional permission to eat.

Meal Planning

We realize some of you may just want to jump to the next section because the phrase "meal planning" has become synonymous with dieting or the new "plan." It is not uncommon for people to have cycles that include periods of time with meticulous meal planning when they are on The Plan, followed by periods of time when they barely go to the store, have little food in the house, and just wing it hour by hour. What we are advocating for in this book is neither of these extremes—you might think of it as a sweet middle path. If you have a long history with diets and prescriptive meal plans, it can really suck the joy out of this part of food caretaking. And sometimes it's even triggering because it is so reminiscent of your dieting days. When it comes to Body Trust and food caretaking, we want you to center pleasure and satisfaction.

First, let's talk about inspiration. Food caretaking can feel like a boring, monotonous job, especially when it's been more about perfecting food instead of what is sounding good to you. What inspires you to eat the foods you eat? Where do you get your inspiration from? Some people flip through food magazines for meal ideas; others look at the store specials, sales, and weekly deals. Going to a farmers market and seeing the seasonal produce can bring to mind a dish or recipe you like and want to re-create. Stores like Trader Joe's and Costco provide samples and even do cooking demos. If you have a collection of cookbooks, you could spend a few hours once a month looking through them and making a list of the recipes you feel drawn to, noting the cookbook and page number. This list can be referenced before you go to the grocery store. Pick a few recipes that sound good for the week and make your shopping list.

Another idea is to make a Favorite Foods list. Put aside your binary categories of good/bad, right/wrong, healthy/unhealthy, etc., and just make a list of the foods you like to eat. Putting it on the list doesn't mean you are committing to eating it! You are just making a list of foods you've enjoyed eating in the past. Think about things you liked as a child. What did you enjoy before you started trying to control and perfect food? It can help to think about breakfast and lunch foods as well as snacky things, even though you can eat these foods any time of day. In your mind's eye, walk yourself through the grocery aisles and add things to your list. Then think about your favorite restaurant dishes. Get specific. Not just Thai food, but what Thai dishes do you like? Not just cookies, but whose cookies? Whose French fries? What kind of pizza? Thick or thin crust? Red or white sauce? Toppings? Frozen? It is all welcome here. You will adjust the list over time, deleting things you try and realize aren't doing it for you anymore. And adding things you discover along the way. Eventually, you can start experimenting with the foods that are less scary and incorporate scarier foods over time to help rebuild trust. One at a time if that is best for you.

With some time and attention, you'll have more ideas to help you make your shopping list and have options on hand for the week. We are not suggesting that you know on Sunday what you will eat on Thursday or that you plan out every single meal. What we want you to have are some ideas for how you will meet your food needs throughout the week. If you have to plan, purchase, and prepare the food all on the same day, it will likely feel overwhelming. You'll throw your hands in the air and either skip the meal or settle for something that isn't satisfying, which is something we all do at times. Let's just not make a habit of it.

It is no joke that this is time consuming. And it's hard to add into your life if it hasn't been there before. This practice, however you end up working with it, is about acknowledging your need to eat regularly. Which is, in essence, acknowledging your humanity.

MEAL PREPARATION AND COOKING

You might not feel very skilled in the kitchen, and you wouldn't be alone in that. Most of us don't learn how to prepare and cook food in school, so if you didn't grow up cooking with the adults in your life, following a recipe can feel overwhelming. You might not know how to use a knife or prep the ingredients in a recipe. The good news is there are plenty of things on the market today that require little to no preparation and are pretty simple to heat up and eat. Don't make it harder than it needs to be, especially when you are just starting out. Remember, fed is best.

If you are interested in learning how to cook, we highly recommend YouTube videos! You can find a YouTube tutorial on just about everything these days (thank you, content creators). Wondering how to cut an onion? Or what it means to julienne carrots? Or how in the world people get the seeds out of a pomegranate without having juice all over everything? Look it up on YouTube, and in a matter of minutes you'll find a short video that shows you how. Dishes will not always come out great the first time you make them. And guess what? You will get better with practice. The more you practice, the more comfortable you become in the kitchen. Tell a friend who cooks a lot that you are wanting to learn how to cook and ask if you can help them cook sometime. Perhaps they have a specific dish you love that you want to learn how to make. Or check out your local community college or food banks, as they sometimes offer basic cooking classes. With time, experimentation, and practice, we are confident you'll be able to find a handful of dishes you can prepare and enjoy eating!

Recommendations for Moving Forward

Your relationship with food is essential to life. Your experiences with food and eating since birth have paved the way for how you nourish yourself today. We want you to take into consideration the truth of your experiences beyond the constructs and constraints of society and the way diet culture encourages you to prioritize the rules of another plan over your own needs and desires. There's a lot of distance between the rigidity and perfectionism of prescriptive plans and the fuck-it-fuck-you-fuck-diet-culture plan. Body Trust asks you to stay out of these binaries so you can arrive in the land of discernment. Here are some recommendations to help you move forward and recommit to being an eater:

> **Reclaim your right to eat and enjoy food.** Every body at every weight deserves adequate nourishment every day. You do not have to earn it. Work on accepting that your body requires food as part of the contract of being alive. Nothing you do gets you out of this contract, no matter how hard you try. And while this coping has served you in some ways, over time your body has suffered, your life has become small, and the world misses out on what makes you *you*.

Neutralize food and eating. Make the apple morally equivalent to the chocolate bar, the fish and chips equivalent to the salad with grilled salmon, etc. Lay aside the food rules so you can begin to connect to your own truth. Remember, you do not gain or lose weight, nor do you become healthy or unhealthy, from one meal or one day of eating.

Eat regularly throughout the day. Most of the meals we eat last no more than three to four hours before our bodies need fuel, sometimes even less. If it has been more than five hours since your last meal, your body needs fuel regardless of whether or not you feel hungry. Set a timer as a reminder to eat, if needed. Once you start consistently feeding yourself, your hunger cues are more likely to come back online. Work to see hunger as a welcome body signal telling you it's time to eat. Reduce habits used to silence hunger, like skipping breakfast, chewing gum, smoking, or drinking tea, water, or diet soda.

Cultivate the ability to observe what happens without judgment. Notice the beliefs that arise about eating a particular food. Investigate where these beliefs come from. Tell your food policing voice(s) to take a back seat. Body Trust isn't about always doing what you (or they) think is the right thing. It's about trusting you'll be okay regardless of what happens. And there will most certainly be another opportunity to practice.

Remember the habituation effect. The more you are exposed and allowed to eat foods you've previously forbidden, the more you tire of them. They lose their elevated status. This is why leftovers are less appealing on day three and why kids who are allowed to eat sweets don't go overboard when sugary foods are presented to them. Without habituation, food remains exciting and scary, and the belief that we must be controlled remains locked in place. If you don't go through the phase of eating foods to habituate to them, it will be hard to transform your relationship with food.

Pay attention to your food while you are eating. It is common for people to eat while doing other things, like working, driving, reading, or watching TV. When you are first recovering from an eating disorder, it might even be helpful to eat with distractions to help reduce the anxiety you feel when you think you shouldn't be eating. So we aren't suggesting you make this a hard-and-fast rule. If and when possible, pause to notice the colors, textures, aromas, and flavors. Do you like it? Does it taste good? If you don't like something, get curious about why you are eating it. In the moment, you may need to make do with what you've prepared or what's available because you don't have time or money to make or get something else. But make a mental note that the food/meal was not enjoyable for you. Pause every now and then to check in with your body to assess how full you are and how much more you need to eat to feel satisfied. Remember: C- work.

Look and listen for attitude changes. Knowing when you are full is not always about experiencing the feeling of fullness, especially when you are recalibrating and trying to connect with the subtler signs that indicate that you've had enough to eat. When you start to tune in and pay attention, you might notice you are losing interest in the food, eating more slowly, not getting as much pleasure from the food, or taking more pauses between bites for conversation or to attend to other things like checking your emails or digging back into work. You might forget about the food and not really think about taking another bite until you see the food again. When we are getting full, there can be a subtle attitude shift from "this is so yummy" to "sigh . . . this is work."

If/when it is hard to say good-bye to food, provide reassurance. Many people experience mixed and intense emotions when your head or your heart wants more than your body is telling you that you need. Food can be a very reliable source of pleasure and comfort—it certainly doesn't talk back—and finishing a snack or meal can be a real bummer. Some folks experience incredible sadness at the end of an eating episode. It can be reassuring to say to yourself, "I will eat again soon . . . when I'm ready." Remember, this work is about healing from chronic expectations of deprivation. Reminders that you will eat again and regularly can be very soothing.

Think about what you want your last bite to be. Making a conscious decision about what you want your last bite to be is a helpful concept we learned from the book *Intuitive Eating*, by Evelyn Tribole and Elyse Resch. When you begin to recognize that you've had enough to eat, think about how many more bites you need to feel satisfied and what foods/flavors you want in that last bite. After you take your last bite, reinforce your decision to stop eating by making a symbolic gesture—push the plate away, put your utensils and napkin down, push back from the table, etc. (It feels important to clarify that we are *not* talking about the diet strategy of sabotaging your food so you don't eat it!) If you notice those feelings of sadness/grief/loss rising when you take that last bite, think of them like a wave that will move through you. Of course, you may grieve the putting down of a coping mechanism that has been steadfast. The wave will have a peak of intensity that will crest and subside. If the desire lingers on, take that as a sign you really need it and eat.

Take risks with your eating so you can learn from your experiences. Every eating episode is an opportunity to practice awareness, connection, and choice. Notice what happens when you eat this versus that. Notice the difference between what you think will happen and what really happens. For example, you might look at a menu in a restaurant and feel really drawn to order a certain item. And then this fear kicks in that you won't be satisfied with it. You can listen to the fear and order the thing that feels more comfortable. Or you can take a risk, order the food you feel called to order, and see what happens. Nothing will change just by reading about it. It takes practice and patience. There's no getting it wrong. Every experience is an opportunity to learn what does and does not work for you.

Notice how long your meals last—how much time passes before you are hungry again. In addition to how much you eat, the combination of foods eaten at one time—the meal mix—influences how long the meal will sustain you. Meals with a combination of fat, protein, fiber, and carbohydrate sustain us for much longer periods of time than meals consisting of mostly fruits and vegetables. People who complain about being hungry all the time may not be eating a meal mix that allows for longer satiety. For example, a bowl of cereal might sustain you for two hours, while scrambled eggs with buttered toast sustains you for three to four hours. This is not to say that one choice is better than the other. One of many factors to consider when making decisions about what and how much to eat is "How long do I need this meal to sustain me?"

Write yourself some permission slips. You may remember that when you were a child, your parents had to sign permission slips for you to participate in school activities. We've found that many of our clients benefit from writing permission slips for the things they want to experiment with and practice. If you feel drawn to this idea, grab a few slips of paper, write down some statements, and

post them where you will see them or keep them in your pocket.
Here are a few examples:

> Jen can eat cookies after dinner.

> Angela is allowed to order what she wants in restaurants.

> Shay has permission to throw food out when she doesn't like it.

> It is okay to take seconds when you're still hungry or just want more because it tastes good.

> Scout has permission to rest. They don't have to go to the gym every day.

Experiment with *yes, no,* and *not now.* Playing around with these three phrases when you are making decisions about your life is a critical part of claiming body sovereignty. Your body is yours. Your preferences are yours. Your time is yours. You don't have to eat things you do not like. You don't have to do things you don't want to do when you are already beyond your capacity. And you don't always have to say yes to food to say "fuck you" to diet culture. We want you to start to celebrate your yeses, honor your noes, and also experiment with the phrase "not now." Saying "not now" is a way you can tend to the part of you that fears deprivation, that doesn't trust you to eat foods you enjoy because when you've said no in the past, it meant never. You may feel drawn to a dessert on the menu, but after checking in with your body and noticing you are pretty full, you decide to say "not now" to the dessert. In this example, you could order and take the dessert home to enjoy later. Or you could make a mental note to go back and have it another time. And here's something that might feel really radical: if you notice there's a dessert you really want to have, order it up front and ask the server to bring it with the rest of your meal. That way you can navigate your hunger and eating, and include bites of dessert along the way. There's no one right way to do something. You can think outside the box. Break the rules and see what happens. You'll learn more about yourself, your needs and desires, what satisfies you, and what doesn't do the trick.

We hope this chapter offers some ways to rethink and reframe your eating. As you practice the various concepts we've shared in this chapter, we promise it will get easier and you won't have to think about your habits so much. That's why we practice. If you think back on any new skill you are trying to learn, like driving a car, it is awkward and clunky at first and you have to think about every single little thing you are doing. But with time and practice, not doing it becomes harder than doing it. Lean on those foundations of Body Trust. Keep the lens wide. Work the edges of your comfort zone. Be gentle with yourself. And perhaps most important, remember C- work.

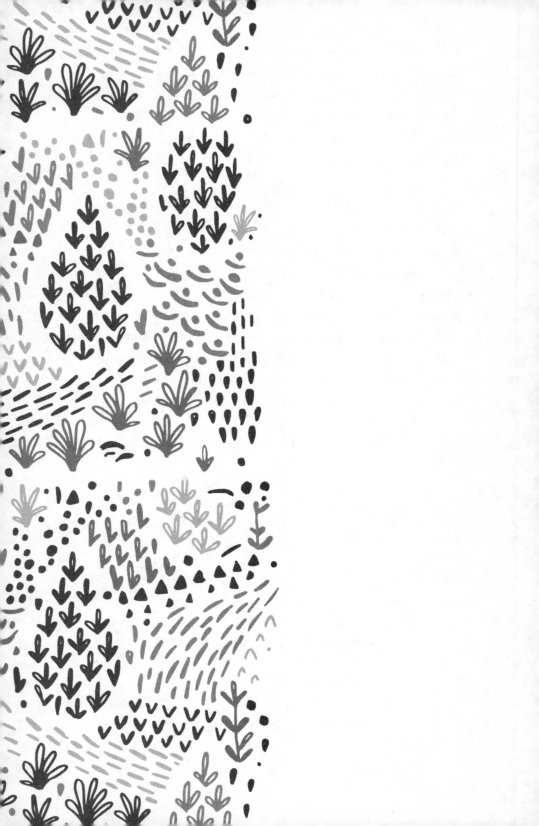

CHAPTER 6

What Does Grief Have to Do with It?

In my healing I am also mourning.

—LAMA ROD OWENS[1]

What role does grief play as you work to heal your relationship with food and body? Some of you may be just coming into the idea that it isn't your fault that trying to change your body hasn't worked. This is sometimes where the grief lives—in understanding that you have not failed, but have been failed. And that your focus on "bettering" yourself was prescribed and barely chosen. Now that you are considering living a life in relationship with your body without the false rescue of weight loss, there is probably a lot arising in you.

As you shift away from body blame and control, what might you be grieving?

* The illusion of control

* Time lost

* The loss of coping

∗ Your eating disorder

∗ The thin ideal or the big reveal

∗ Money spent

∗ Misdirected energy

∗ Acceptance of others' bullshit narratives about your body

∗ The settling you've done in relationships, family, clothes, ambition, and your bucket list

∗ The prioritization of anti-fatness and moving up the body hierarchy instead of living your truth

∗ That you've been colluding and caused harm (especially if you are a provider)

∗ The loss of relationships that can't support this healing process

∗ The things you lose when you allow for change

As we move further into the reckoning, we likely are also grieving the loss of what has been a foundational coping mechanism. We know that for many of us, our coping operates as a container, holding anxiety, uncertainty, and shame, distracting and directing it to the one problem we wish we could solve. Our disordered eating does something for us. It may quiet wanting, needing, or longing so you can continue to drive forward. It may have allowed you to survive adversity and traverse mountains while it held aspects of your life that you were not yet able to reckon with and heal from. We may want to stand back for a moment and admire this way of getting through difficulty, and be grateful that our psyche can work in these layered ways. Author Savala Nolan speaks to this awareness:

> *Even with the money to pay a trainer's exorbitant fees, my body*
> *will never comply enough, will always be subject to the harms*

of fatphobia, some of which can be empirically measured and some of which cannot. This is why I think it comes down to the body. Whatever else life hands you, your body fundamentally protects and shields you, or is fundamentally a target. So I turn to my privilege for help, I entreat it for assistance, but often it just continues playing, capricious and self-absorbed; that's its prerogative, that's its very essence. No matter how privileged I get, with my fat-ish, Black, female body, the burdens are always nipping at my heels. The body is inevitable. It can't be masked. For better or worse, the body endures.[2]

What you may be sitting with is a bit of an *oh shit* kind of moment. What is your life to be without body obsession, disordered eating, dieting, food plans? Many of us have felt highly distracted by the presence of body and/or food obsession, if not downright obsessed. As we have talked about previously, it may be scary to approach it and choose to reckon with this and consider letting go.

What is healing if not also a grief process? What is reckoning if not informed by what wasn't, what should have been, or by what we have lost or will absolutely lose soon enough? When we divorce healing from self-improvement, we are steered toward making deeper meaning. We can say there is something that has been lost in the pursuit of the perfect body. There have been parts stifled, orphaned, and buried in The Hustle. There have been essential parts of being human that have been disregarded, disrespected, ignored, and harmed.

Grief is a natural emotional state. It is a part of us, something our beings undertake and simply do. It is hard. It has otherworldly qualities. Grief is a path toward reclamation because it is a deepening of process, an honoring. It allows us to discover more about ourselves. It is a necessary catharsis. To grieve is to be alive. To be human. And because it is a deeply human experience, it benefits from being ritualized and having space held for it.

A Body Trust participant talked about it this way:

> *It is hard to accept my body. I thought I had done that, but not really. I still have vague plans and use clothes to keep me in check. As I journey through some of the old beliefs I hold about myself, I am sad, angry, grieving. Grief is pretty big for me right now, which means I am right on track.*
>
> *My body, my intuition, knows these societal ideas about the body—which I have internalized—have been wrong all this time. Tapping into the truth is releasing the pain.*

This may be a time to remember that most of us were indoctrinated into societal constructs that led us to hustle for the perfect body. Now that you've read more of this book, we wonder what else you remember about the first time you learned that your body is a problem. What had to be sublimated, disremembered, protected, or lost when you became the problem? What got relegated to the shadows, made suspect or distrusted? Which parts of you have you learned not to trust because they did not meet expectations? We grieve when we have been wronged and we also grieve when we were wrong. It is all grief. It is all ours to move through.

Grief arises in the dissonance between wanting to believe we can control our bodies and coming to terms with the biological reality that we cannot, that there are complex regulatory systems at play that will kick in to restore your body to the place it naturally wants to be. We can spend our entire lives chasing the fantasy and blaming ourselves when another plan doesn't work . . . yet again. Or we can begin to fully let the truth sink in and experience loss. Attending to the grief that accompanies this loss is part of the healing process. You may be familiar with the stages of grief that Elisabeth Kübler-Ross described in 1969: denial, anger, bargaining, depression, and acceptance.[3] What most people do not know is that Kübler-Ross's stages were named to bring understanding to "describe the process patients go through as they come to terms with their terminal illness."[4] The stages of grief were later applied more widely. People who are living with chronic illnesses, and life-changing diagnoses such as cancer, multiple sclerosis, lupus, epilepsy, etc. benefit from allowing space for grief to emerge.

We ask you, as we begin to talk about the layers of grief, to please divest yourself from thinking of grieving as a linear process. Expect a mess that switches or layers themes with fervor. Much like when we give way to flight when we board a plane, or trust the wheels of the bike as we begin to descend a hill, we let grief move us. Grief is not ever simplified. But there are themes in this human, natural process. Let's look at them and consider how they relate to our relationship with our bodies:*

Denial

When you first heard about Body Trust, we guess that there may have been a part of you that said, *"No, no, no, no, no,"* or "I can't trust my body." We want to stop time, hold the hope, grip on to the illusion of control and the familiar.

In this phase, people experience avoidance, confusion that may give way to elation, shock, and fear. You may find yourself continuing to restrict your food despite acknowledging that sustained weight loss is impossible for most people. Or you may cling to a belief that maintaining weight loss will happen when you find the right plan. You continue to look to outside experts to tell you what, when, and how much to eat. You remain detached from your body and navigate life through the language of "food and fat" instead of your hunger, feelings, or lived experience.

When considering all this, it's common for people to feel pulled back into the familiar territory of diet culture—to wander away from

---

* We were so grateful to be introduced to Jeanne Courtney and her paper "Size Acceptance as a Grief Process: Observations from Psychotherapy with Lesbian Feminists," *Journal of Lesbian Studies* 12, no. 4 (2008): 347–63. Her work inspired our thoughts on this and gave us language to build on.

and then return to this work. Body Trust Provider Meredith Noble writes: "We forget that dieting has been a fair-weather friend. We remember the intoxicating joy of our weight loss successes, but forget our misery when the scale is higher than we want it to be, the pain of bingeing to the point of feeling unwell, or the despair of realizing we're starving but have already eaten our maximum number of calories for the day."[5]

When you find yourself feeling drawn to another plan to restrict, restrain, or control food and your body, the first thing to do is notice what's pulling you back in. Did you recently see a friend who is in the honeymoon phase of their diet? Is there an event happening that you have anxiety about? Are there other areas of your life where you feel like you don't have control?

And then remember your lived experience with these plans. How long do they usually last? What do you like about them? What don't you like about them? Body Trust participant L. W. shared the following with us about the pull of the plans:

> There is a freedom in letting go of all of the shoulds. There is a lightness in that, even as my body grows heavier. I look at the communities I am a part of, and look toward helping to create change, knowing this journey of leaving behind my obsessions with food and my weight will create space for that work. On hard days, the energy that keeps me from falling back into diet/wellness culture is currently anger. I'm furious with all of the energies that have kept me preoccupied with my weight and I channel that "fuck you" vibe into telling diet/wellness culture to fuck off. Is that my forever feeling? I don't think so. It is a feeling that needs to move on through; I envision a future where tough days are met simply with kindness and understanding and an anchoring in knowing what my body truly needs.

Anger

"Why? Why? Why?!!!!!" In this phase of grief, we experience feelings like frustration, irritation, anxiety, anger, rage, envy, and resentment. You may rely on familiar patterns of soothing/coping or move into a period of self-loathing/neglect/harm. The continued belief that there is a right way to eat will lead to the pathologizing of any eating, whether it's driven by your physical and/or emotional needs.

It is not unusual in the reckoning process for anger to come more easily than grief or sadness. Weight loss and cosmetic fitness industries make money off your internally directed anger and frustration, but they of course are part of the reason you believed you needed them in the first place. Instead of directing the anger inward, we can begin to shift it toward the systems and institutions that uphold anti-fat bias. Anger has a way of showing us the way. It can kick the reckoning process into high gear because it has the power of lifesaving energy that tells us where our edges are and what we deeply care about. We often return to this piece by the poet David Whyte:

> *Anger is the deepest form of compassion, for another, for the world, for the self, for a life, for the body, for a family and for all our ideals, all vulnerable and all, possibly about to be hurt. Stripped of physical imprisonment and violent reaction, anger is the purest form of care, the internal living flame of anger always illuminates what we belong to, what we wish to protect and what we are willing to hazard ourselves for.*[6]

It's in this phase of grief that we work to give an external focus to the anger and self-blame we are feeling. We get mad at the physical education curriculum that stole our love for movement, the dance teacher who fat-shamed us, the medical establishment that's colluded with diet culture to dupe us into an unnecessary lifelong hustle.

Performance consultant Staci Jordan Shelton says, "Before the truth can set you free, you have to recognize what lies are holding you hostage."[7] What lies are holding you hostage? In what ways have you been harmed by diet culture? In your reckoning, you may notice heat rising in your chest, your heart beating faster, your face reddening. You may feel the urge to scream. Find ways to let yourself feel and express the anger: write it out and throw it in the flames, scream (into a pillow if you must), find a friend willing to hold space to help get it up and out of you, go on a rant. Pound the earth. Put on music and dance.

We benefit from making public (or external) our frustrations. How do you know what you feel? Make a list of your complaints. Let it flow. You may come from a culture that honors the art of kvetching or welcomes the public lament. Maybe your people (or the overarching culture) have silenced this, calling it whining. These expressions are essential. Our self-editing can move in tandem with our self-surveillance. "Listen: That's too much to say, eat, feel. People like me do not have a right to complain, eat, take up space." *No.* That's not it. The silencing of the lament is the silencing of your truth and access to the flow of your emotion. Overarching positivity and overcontrol of mindset is a denial of the complexity of emotional experience and the politicized nature of our lives. Where your emotions live is an expression of your being. To move forward together, we must be in touch with what we can no longer tolerate.

Body Trust participant Angeline P. says this about her reckoning process:

> *I was so angry. I hated fatphobia, diet culture, every asshole who's ever said anything negative or nasty about my body. I hated clothing stores, uncomfortable chairs, my family, my exes, well-meaning fatphobes who couldn't repress playing "help the fattie" (my name for all the concern trolls who can't resist giving me asinine unsolicited advice). I ate everything I'd told myself was bad and wrong. I had cookies for breakfast*

for weeks. I ate whole pizzas regularly (and still do occasionally). I was boiling mad at myself for being bamboozled by wellness diet, after cleanse, after vegan purity puritanism. I was disgusted with myself for being so horrible to people who I'd deemed less desirable and even less lovable due to my own internalized beauty standards and fat phobia. I was boiling mad for a long time and I still come to a simmer on a regular basis, but I've since learned to externalize and I burn myself out a lot less now.

Eventually, most people begin to fuel this anger into activism. In fact, becoming involved in fat activism—and broader social justice movements—can be an integral part of healing and body reclamation work. More on that later.

Bargaining

When we talk about the various stages of grief, this is the part most people can relate to. In this phase, people are negotiating and postponing the inevitable by finding new rationales to keep dieting instead of opting out of diet culture. You'll hear people say things like, *"I'm just trying to be healthy," "I'll lose XXX pounds and then do this Body Trust thing," "My knees . . ."*

The crux of our grief may live in this paradox. Regardless of your history with disordered eating, it is necessary to reckon with how you are continuing to collude with anti-fatness and diet culture and how that impacts your life. Our participation is never benign, despite our best intentions. Our participation upholds anti-fat bias, allows bullshit to proliferate, and lets the lies about diet culture continue. We may seek a version of health that doesn't truly allow us to release ourselves from The Cycle or experience our wholeness. BTW, one of our favorite ways out of conversations centered around weight loss is from our friend, coach

Rachel Cole. She says, "You know how some people don't talk about politics or religion? Well, I don't talk about dieting." Done and done.

This is where reckoning deepens. You may wander away as you bargain and then return as you keep reading, learning, unlearning, exploring, and reminding yourself of what you already know based on your lived experience . . . that it doesn't work. It doesn't align with your values. And you want something different for yourself, your life, and the world.

You will also come to understand how health care providers' training (and the research they quote) is inseparable from anti-fat bias. As our colleague Deb Burgard has said, it is increasingly evident that health care is basically outsourcing itself to the multibillion-dollar diet industry. You may begin backing away from anyone who is profiting from your cycle of shame and deprivation.

You will notice there are people in your life who cannot or will not understand Body Trust. Their fears and judgments do not invalidate your truth or need to engage in a healing process. The fork in the road is uncomfortable. And healing includes knowing your truth and following it for a while to see where it takes you. What is the point of anything else?

We wonder if you can acknowledge that The Hustle for the perfect body is holding you back from doing things you could really do now. And how The Hustle has reinforced a sense of failure, self-loathing, and distrust in yourself, which has impacted how you engage with the world. Your relationship with yourself is what is in need of repair, not you, and certainly not your body. What is needed for repair is respect for the truth, an end to gaslighting, and a building of trust through small, consistent steps over time. No grand gestures. Just showing up again and again. Doing C- work. And letting go of what's no longer your truth.

Depression

In her paper titled "Size Acceptance as a Grief Process," Jeanne Courtney says "preparatory depression is necessary to facilitate acceptance of a loss.

It is about facing the sad fact that a fat-phobic, misogynist world is not an easy place to live."[8] In this phase of grief, allow yourself to lean into and feel the sadness. Find a few people in your life who can sit with you in your pain without constantly trying to fix it or telling you not to be sad.

When we talk about depression as a phase here, we are talking about the challenge of letting go of things that aren't working. Sadness can arise in response to a feeling of futility, a lack of knowledge about what to do next. This is a stage of reckoning and of acknowledging that going back may not be an option, though going forward may not feel wholly possible yet, either. Chronic patterns of dieting and disordered eating lead to disconnection from our inner landscape and our emotions, so you may not be sure what is okay to root into. Sadness can be a vehicle that reminds us of our depth of feeling and allows us to connect to the deeper process of grief. L. W., a Body Trust participant, shared this about their own process:

> I had always sensed a deep anger in myself. It came out in judgment of others, in high anxiety, in being controlling. I was furious that my food had been restricted from the time I was a child but also furious that I couldn't seem to get my shit together and solve the problem of my body. I have had multiple "health professionals" tell me some variation of "but you're so smart, how did you get like this? I'm sure you'll figure it out." As if my body size has anything to do with my intelligence. My anger has always been contained and turned inward. Reckoning has included conceding that the way my parents handled food and my body were abusive (impact over intentions) and that the negative messages/values they instilled in me were just plain wrong and ignorant. Reckoning has also included the knowledge that I will never, ever fit societal beauty standards and I have to practice radical acceptance there. I do grieve that I have never been considered "hot" (generally speaking and not including my lovely husband), and that I

have never experienced the rites of passage that many young
women have, for good or ill.

Body Trust has taught me that my body deserves compas-
sion and kindness and a recognition that it is always doing
the best it can. This has allowed my well of compassion to
grow much deeper, and I am able to extend it to others as well
as to myself. In general I am less angry and more patient, and
more forgiving of human foibles. I feel confident and righteous
in terms of being assertive about my accommodation needs
and setting boundaries. My body shame is all but eliminated,
and I feel freer to show up as I am, wherever I go.

Please know that if you have felt disconnected from your body
for a long time, and/or feel overwhelmed just thinking about this,
you do not have to be all in or go it alone. Working with someone
who specializes in somatic therapy can help you learn ways to gently
access sensations and build distress tolerance over time. We also recommend following and learning from fat positive providers and activists who inspire and lift you up and remind you of your inherent
value and worth.

Acceptance

The idea of acceptance is often misinterpreted as the "fuck it" plan, but
there's a difference between letting go and giving up. Think about that
for a second. How does your body respond when you think about letting
go versus giving up?

Giving up feels like failure. There is a sense of frustration and/or
defeat. It can reinforce some less than great ideas we hold about ourselves—we are not enough, not as good as so-and-so, etc. Sometimes we
give up to protect ourselves and walk away unscathed, but often it feels
unfinished—like there is something to return to.

Letting go has a different energy about it. Letting go roots into truth. More like, *This isn't serving me and I'm walking away. No one knows my truth better than me. I'm laying this down to make room for something else. This is the path, even if I don't like it.* Wellness coach Linda Tucker told us:

> *The reckoning looks like me collapsing to the floor and cry-ing or wailing against the hard edges of the truth . . . that there is no control, no certainty, and no way to avoid feeling my feelings. It's a total surrender. It's a point of exhaustion, where I can no longer hold up the weight on my shoulders, even though I may still desperately WANT to. It feels like a giv-ing up of sorts . . . but in letting go, I am given rest and respite as I lie on the ground.*

In this stage, you're further along in your divestment from diet cul-ture. The opinions and actions of others do not take center stage. Your feelings about your body are more neutral—you want more and dif-ferent for yourself. You want your life to feel like yours now, not XX pounds from now. You'll be less drawn toward external prescriptions for the right way to occupy and care for your body. You take risks to explore what kind of eating patterns work best for you and lean toward pleasure and satisfaction.

It doesn't mean you won't flirt with other stages, as grief is not lin-ear and is often most intense in the beginning. Some use the metaphor of waves crashing ashore to describe grief. When the loss is new, the waves of grief come often, they are intense and seemingly unrelenting. Time, along with allowing feelings, changes grief. The waves become less intense and more spread out. You'll have more buoyancy when they do come. We learn. We adjust. We change. You can be trusted to grow.

Grief is not an individualized experience, though it often plays out within us as if it is. We talked earlier about the benefits of the public lament. During 2020, there was a rise in conversations about collective grief as we weathered a pandemic along with a political uprising in response to the murders of Black people by police. We may also acknowledge that unprocessed grief takes a toll on us as individuals but also permeates the souls of families, communities, and countries, giving rise to the harm of oppression and public denial of harm.

The grief you experience around this work will vary depending on your size, gender, race, ethnicity, ability, and more. Grief may be best held in groups of people who most understand your experience. Having spaces that allow for the ritual or processing of grief that are specific to identity are essential.

An individualized focus alone is not enough for healing, especially for an illness born of a sick world. As much as this work is about moving the problem focus outside of your body, our grief work must be about acknowledging the depth and universal aspects of our grief. We are grieving more than just what hasn't worked for us personally. Our grief is part of a lineage for the way that dominant systems have marginalized vast groups of people. White dominant culture does not feed any of us; it starves us while we hustle.

Grief can feel as though it is slipping through our fingers because we do not often believe we are equipped to hold something so unresolvable. It accumulates in us as we live. Some of it never fades. We, in order to become a collective that desires healing, must learn to live with grief as a companion. We will not resolve all the harm we have done to each other or ourselves in our lifetime. We will continue to witness and participate in harm. Our choices will not always be clean. We can increase our ability to weather this and arrive in relationships leading with empathy, curiosity, and trust in the lived experience of others. We hope Body Trust is helping you see your body story more clearly and that you feel less like hiding your lived experience.

Kari V. shared part of her story with us:

Restriction led to closet eating, and further shame was introduced when I was molested by a family member. No chance for justice was allowed after the crime happened, so my physical safety and complete disconnection with my body was in full swing by the time I was thirteen. I remember feeling a constant hollowness in my center and a tightness around my throat and I moved through middle school trying to fill the hollowness by bingeing, then hoping the food would somehow latch on to all the pain and sorrow inside which could be completely excised with an ipecac chaser. The euphoria and overall numbness brought about by the exorcism of bingeing and purging became my shameful secret, which continued on and off until I was able to move away from my family and live on my own. The reckoning phase of healing for me has been looking back to understand that so much of my relationship with my body has been about wanting to change the past. Working through the rage of how I was valued more for my body than for who I am from those who should have loved me still comes up at times today. When it comes up, I face it head on and use the tools I have used through twenty-five years of therapy to work on changing the future and forgiving the past.

Because grief can feel so big and overwhelming, we have found that creating a physical reminder in the form of an intentional space, an altar, or a shrine to your grief and change process can keep the work alive and remind you it's real, that you are real, and that this process is important to you. When we asked some of our program participants what they would add to an altar they said:

* A stuffed broken bear to remind myself of self-soothing through the grief process.

* A picture of myself in seventh grade. What I see now is a vibrant young lady who looks like all the other girls in her class. When I was that age, I remember distinctly seeing that picture and being horrified by my size. I grieve for what I could not see then and for all the time I spent in heartache wishing for a different body.

* A replica of the Venus of Willendorf or something similar. This image stirs grief in me because it reminds me that societal love for these bodies has been lost and how much we have lost because of it.

* A beautiful leaf, dry and brittle, to represent the cycle of shedding and letting go.

* My old journal from the time I was struggling the most with food and body. I sometimes look back at it and remember how sad and painful it was to be in that place, which allows for both grief and self-compassion.

* Fuckin' ass spirulina. That shit made me cry x 100. Release.

* A picture of a child twirling in circles. I remember doing this as a young child before I dissociated for so long.

* Buttons, to remind me of all the buttons that would not close.

* Photos of my elders, especially my mom and her mom, whose bodies were like mine and whose bodies I loathed as much as my own.

* A stone to symbolize my body's connection to the earth, something blue to symbolize my body's connection to the sky, and a mirror to remind me of how easy it is to forget and get lured back.

Invite it in. Give the grief a seat. Feed it. Make it a practice. Lama Rod Owens says,

> We have to make mourning our main practice right now. The wounds are deep, old, and pervasive. We have been wounded by many systems of power and abuse, including capitalism. Wounds just don't disappear. We have to do the work of touching into the hurt and allowing the energy to rise in spaciousness as we experience and release the energy. It's hard work. It's not supposed to be easy. If we want to be healed, we have to work.

Nothing is a guarantee. Including our bodies and our health. We make a practice of allowing for change again and again—not liking it but not controlling it. Grieving it and being true to what it is alive in us and asking for attention. Recognizing and allowing grief can be part of our practice.

I Woke Up Like That

by Angela Braxton-Johnson

I don't know if I wanna be fat
Right now
But I woke up like that

So how
In this world do I cope

With trauma
Using food as dope
Diet fads and societal drama
Expending hope

Choked up
Judged by my chocolate skin-tone

Locked up
Sentenced as unworthy
Crowded and alone

Journeying home
To Myself
My Fabulousness
My Beauty
My Uniqueness
My Truthness
My Surviving-no-matter-what-happens-ness
My Being-fearfully-and-wonderfully-made-ness

By transforming grace my greatness resounds
Confounding oblivious, ignorant
Non-supporters of Abundance
And Fatness
And Melanin
And Girls

Loving and accepting me
Just as I am

Female
Unveiled
With my round curvy shell
Fat and Black

Yeah
I woke up like that[9]

CHAPTER 7

Ending the Hustle

*My perfectionism arose as an attempt to gain safety and
support in my dangerous family. Perfection is a self-persecutory
myth. I do not have to be perfect to be safe or loved in the
present. I am letting go of relationships that require perfection.*[1]

—PETE WALKER, author of *Complex PTSD: From Surviving to Thriving*

Systems teach us a hustle to survive them. They do not care if you are tired, how able-bodied you may or may not be, economically devastated, recovering, or historically marginalized. The same ideals that belittle us turn around and teach us to strive to become better. Our nervous systems become accustomed to what systems demand and subsequently normalize. Our coping is necessary in these systems. The striving, competing, bootstrapping, and hustling all become part of what "needs to happen" to be enough, interesting, valuable, and successful. Some of us do this simply to survive the hierarchy. Some do this to uphold internalized dominance. Most often it is both.

There are elephants in the room we can only vaguely see but most certainly can feel. Our culture buzzes around them, bending and shaping themselves to make room but rarely, if ever, stopping to say, "What the fuck is this?" or naming all the constructs and cultural ideals within our systems that fuel The Hustle. In this chapter, we will be unpacking some ideas about shame and worthlessness that interrupt our presence with ourselves—and others—and keep us feeling fragmented and less than whole and worthy.

The rubber meets the road when you want this new paradigm and you still really want to lose some weight. Why wouldn't you, given the culture we live in? Everything we've been taught about weight is inaccurate. Everything we've been taught about how much control we have over our size is also likely wrong. The dissonance this creates can certainly put us in touch with a feeling of shame. However, scapegoating and rejecting Body Positivity, Health at Every Size (HAES), and/or Fat Liberation discourse are not emotionally honest. Instead, name the shitstorm of feelings that accompanies acknowledging that you have been duped by weight loss culture. Be frustrated by the way weight loss hope cyclically returns to your life and lets you down. Bang down the doors of all the "integrative weight loss approaches" and let them know they aren't so different. Tell everyone to stop colluding with the part of your mind that believes parts of you are unacceptable.

You do not have to agree with everything in the body liberation movement to support it, but if you are here, you must include all bodies. In order to include all bodies, we must use language to question and denounce the levity we bring to weight loss conversations. Understand that living in a fat body in our society is significantly and consistently challenging and frequently harmful. When weight loss is casually laid on the table, weight stigma and anti-fat bias continue, and eating disorders persist. If your feminism is to be intersectional, then know that our weight discussions have roots in racism, ableism, sizeism, and a binary view of gender. In fact, as Sirius Bonner writes in her essay "A Brief History of the Fat Acceptance Movement,"

> [A] lack of understanding or belief in a shared struggle, or what we might now call an intersectional analysis, meant

*that many fat folks were shut out of fat activism. Let's take
a look at the impact of race as an example. Many activists
associated with NAAFA (National Association to Advance Fat
Acceptance) and other mainstream branches of the movement tended to be single-issue activists; they were reluctant
to incorporate other social justice issues into their activism
as they thought it would detract from their goals. While fat,
many of these activists lived with the privileges of being white,
heterosexual, cisgender, middle or upper class, and/or American; they had very little incentive to incorporate other struggles into their activism. This resulted in the voices of people
of color, among others, being left out of the mainstream fat acceptance movement. At the same time, they also assumed that
communities of color were more accepting of fatness and so
this kind of activism was unnecessary in those communities.
Their lack of intersectional analysis meant that they did not
understand the ways that fatphobia showed up across racial
groups. Similarly, they did not understand that fat folk of color
experienced compounding oppression from white culture for
not being white or thin.*

If we tried to make this light and easy, as it is commonly represented
in media and in lunchroom conversations, it would include only white,
cis-gender, able-bodied women. This isn't light and easy no matter how
you spin it. As with any other social justice issue, your stance has an impact. And the middle path will not change the world.

Economic systems would crumble if we did this differently. While
we lived through the pandemic and upheaval of 2020, and on the side
worried about weight gain while the collective grief mounted, the weight
loss industry still grossed $71 billion.[2] While we couldn't go in person,
the fitness industry grossed $27 billion in the United States.[3] Cosmetics
and personal care brought in $39 billion,[4] though most of our faces were

partially covered by masks or were visible only via Zoom. We spend our money here, which is fine. But it also is likely inhibiting the analysis of what is indeed valuable for improving the quality of our lives. One of the most profitable things the powers that be could create was to highlight a giant connection between health and weight and then offer solutions that don't work.

When we want to feel well, we are often met with an onslaught of self-improvement strategies. The way concepts of healing are described and understood in the field of nutrition, as well as alternative and complementary medicine circles, are often met with minimal analysis. Leah Lakshmi Piepzna-Samarasinha, author of *Care Work: Dreaming Disability Justice*, says, "Mainstream ideas of 'healing' deeply believe in ableist ideas that you're either sick or well, fixed or broken, and that nobody would want to be in a disabled or sick or mad bodymind. . . . Unsurprisingly and unfortunately, these ableist ideas often carry over into healing spaces that call themselves 'alternative' or 'liberatory.'"[5]

Who do our ideas of health include? And why do we believe in health as a goal when it moves through our society more as a status? When we pursue health to increase our quality of life, why is it that our next thought does not extend to how we improve access and quality of life for all people regardless of health status? Health is an individualized construct and the ammunition raised against those who fail to pursue it "well enough."

Diet culture teaches people to approach the body and food with rigidity and perfectionism. The way society talks about nutrition and health, you'd think one meal or day of eating has the power to heal or kill you. Starting with unrealistic expectations and then being hard on yourself when you can't pull it off are how the weight loss and cosmetic fitness industries make money off your shame.

As we discussed in chapter 5, "Reckoning with Your Eating," when we live in a culture that values food restriction and dietary restraint, it can be hard to know what you are really choosing for yourself and to see how your choices are rooted in a dieting mindset. Before you succumb to shame or hating us, we want to gently remind you it is not your fault that you hold this conditioning. But please also recognize that any of the little intuitions, niggling wonderings, and questioning you've done of this process was your wisdom showing you another possibility . . . another way.

What's wrong with your commitment to health? Nothing. It's just a more complicated construct than culture and capitalism have built. Health is not a place we arrive and stay, but more of an idea. It's not static; our bodies will change throughout our lives because of *life*. We are so scared of not being able to control it. But instead of feeling that, we love nothing more than making it a hobby: talking about health, thinking about health, proselytizing about health, and selling health to one another. It's exhausting once you see it. And there is a word for this: healthism.

Healthism is an ideology that reinforces the pursuit of health as worthy above all things. Healthism recommends perfecting nutrients despite the hypervigilance that it ignites. Healthism diagnoses by sight. Healthism says that a long life is the be-all and end-all and that we have control over lifelong health. Healthism bootstraps and blames, rewarding privilege but calling it discipline and success. Healthism bypasses anti-fat bias that underlies all our health research. Healthism funds so-called obesity research but not eating disorder research unless it centers on small or thin bodies (or tries to fix "obesity"). Healthism says anorexia can occur only in emaciated bodies instead of bodies of all sizes. Healthism has no qualms about gaslighting you as the industry takes your money and bank on your minimized self-regard. Healthism preys on your work ethic, your belief in always striving to do better, and your conflicted ideas about the worthiness of your body. Healthism is everywhere—it's in the atmosphere that we breathe, and it sucks. When asked how Body Trust has helped to see the world differently, Body Trust participant L. W. shared:

I recognize the ways in which the shift I made from diet cul-
ture to an obsession with "wellness" was a shifting that did lit-
tle to create a sense of trust in myself. I have more kindness for
myself and for others. The idea of healthism has shaken much
of my foundation about well-being on a community level.

The impacts of healthism, nutritionism, and ableism are felt and truly harmful, and they are also so woven into the fabric of our so-called values about health that they can be tough to discern. In an article in *Critical Public Health*, Jennifer Brady and her colleagues write, "The term 'nutritionism' has been coined to describe the fixation on nutrients, at the expense of context and experiential knowledge of food and eating, and the resulting 'nutrition confusion' that has confounded people's ideas about what to eat."[6] Nutritionism simultaneously disembodies us while fueling our hustle *and* being quite profitable. It tends to bypass the impacts of food apartheid and supermarket redlining, as well as the impact of oppression, chronic trauma and abuse. The misuse of power and wealth makes food and behavior recommendations for only those who can participate.

Nutritionism has a strong hold on our culture. It seems impossible to get through a day without hearing someone's opinion about what constitutes "healthy eating" because of the dualistic thinking it promotes: if there is a good nutrient, then there must be a bad one. Nutritionism causes unnecessary food worry and makes eating far more complicated than it needs to be. The desire to take care of our food needs often diminishes when we are only focused on eating the "right thing." And if you have a history of chronic dieting or disordered eating, you might feel conflicted about almost every single food available for your consumption. Such a distracting and unnecessary hustle. How is this about health?

This system proliferates on the devaluation of bodies. Fat people, yes, and Black and brown people, disabled people, gender expansive and trans people, women, femmes, and elders. It's obvious and infuriating and there is no valid counterargument to its existence. The hustle that we speak of is about seeing your place in this system and defying the systems that uphold the body hierarchy. Not dedicating your life to hustling away from the parts of living in a human body that may not truly be in our control. As we find that many of us are hustling in response to systemic and inter-personal anti-fat bias, we are doing the same regarding ableism.

Just in case ableism is new to you, here is what we mean: Ableism is the set of policies, practices, norms, and attitudes that devalue and limit the lives of people with developmental, psychiatric, physical, or emotional disability. The disabled lived experience is typically made in-visible through further oppression in a world that doesn't prioritize and understand equitable access and holds nondisabled people as normative while further disabling disabled people due to barriers the dominant culture doesn't address. Unless we are admiring those who defy the odds and do incredible things despite disability instead of understanding that folks with disability are disabled by "normie" culture. The differences in lived experience are a point of othering instead of honoring disabled ex-perience as central to understanding our shared humanity. Here's a basic truth that is missing from our everyday understanding: Sick people have and always will exist. Disabled people have and always will exist. Fat people have and always will exist. If personal and collective conscious-ness considered these lived experiences inherent and normative instead of fringe, what would we hustle for?

Scholar Caleb Luna (@chairbreaker on Instagram) posted a sum-mary of the connections between these intersections titled "On Fat Em-bodiment & Divesting from Constructions of Health." Some of what they offered included:

> Disabled people have let us know that we can become disabled instantaneously through accident or illness: in fact, it is part of life. If we live long enough, we will eventually become dis-abled in some way. The emphasis on health devalues disabled people, whose bodies will never achieve these standards.

Illness is innate to the human condition and many people who structure their lives around diet culture still contract viruses, develop cancers and other conditions. There is no diet or exercise regime that is guaranteed to prevent illness or injury.[7]

The Hustle has asserted that if you play your cards right (cards such as willpower, discipline, mindset, etc.), you will rise above the social constructs designed to profit from—and harm—you, and you will win. And then people will respect you. And then others will look at you and not worry about you based on the sight of you, and then . . . No. None of this happens. And it's not up to you to make it better for only you. This is a broader issue that you exist within. And a broader, less individualist response will change us.

"It's not about self-care—it's about collective care," writes Leah Lakshmi Piepzna-Samarasinha:

Collective care means shifting our organizations to be ones where people feel fine if they get sick, cry, have needs, start late because the bus broke down, move slower, ones where there's food at meetings, people work from home—and these aren't things we apologize for. It is the way we do the work, which centers disabled-femme-of-color ways of being in the world, where many of us have often worked from our sickbeds, our kid beds, or our too-crazy-to-go-out-today beds. Where we actually care for each other and don't leave each other behind. Which is what we started with, right?[8]

Much of what we do in the name of health causes more stress than it relieves. There is so much that happens in healing processes and therapeutic modalities that wants to make your behaviors the problem. This work is about getting the problem narrative outside of you. You are not the problem to solve, though it makes sense that you have tried to solve it through your efforts to change your body. Reminder: It hasn't worked because it doesn't work. Not because you are wrong or have done wrong. Part of this reckoning is recognizing the habitual responses, beliefs, and unprocessed grief that live within you due to the oppressive nature of the world around you, that keep you hustling regardless.

Healing body dissatisfaction/loathing is not necessarily about liking the image of your body. It's not solely about changing the way you see or experience your body. It is very much about turning toward and unraveling the body loathing, shame, and oppression that have turned your body into a thing needing to be altered and improved. This cultural stuff was never yours, though you may feel overrun by it. In *What We Don't Talk About When We Talk About Fat*, author Aubrey Gordon writes: "Its rallying cry, love your body, presumes that our greatest challenges are internal, a poisoned kind of thought about our own bodies. It cannot adapt to those of us who love our bodies, but whose bodies are rejected by those around us, used as grounds for ejecting us from employment, healthcare, and other areas of life."[9]

During our years working in eating disorder treatment, we've come to believe that what we call body image should be fat affirmation work. Unfortunately, and inappropriately, fat affirmation has been considered too political, optional, debatable, or dangerous in therapeutic and eating disorder treatment communities. It is not fringe-y. It is essential. It is an issue of inclusion. Anything else is a denial of both lived experience and ongoing harm. It scaffolds sustainable healing for those suffering from disordered eating, though you would be hard pressed to find a treatment facility with affirming pictures of fat people. Some won't even invest in furniture to fit a variety of body sizes. The eating disorder field is wrong. We haven't been brave enough as a profession to assert this truth. And when we are, we are often silenced by dominant opinions predicated on "research" that doesn't address the conscious and unconscious anti-fat bias that upholds it.

People cannot recover sustainably without addressing the personal and systemic impact of weight stigma and anti-fat bias. Internalized oppression and body shame have to be named not merely as "thinking errors," but as the very real experience of having a body that is subject to othering and pathologizing. Maybe this is why body image work has primarily served only white, cis-gender women. And it hasn't really served them well, either.

Do not tolerate "body image work" that exclusively places the burden of healing upon the individual alone. Marginalized communities know the beauty and necessity of community care. Body image work is a false notion. Our collective commitment to the inclusion of all bodies is where belonging and healing are enacted.

We recommend that you not engage with providers or programs that promote weight change as a way to improve body image. Question them. Clinicians, note that your ability to feel comfortable offering fat affirmation work will be enhanced by exploring your own body story and process. This is essential work, not a specialization.

Let us question what we really want when we speak of body image work. We want freedom for bodies and we want inclusion. We want systemic change and less body shunning, blame, and shame. Shame itself can be a powerful force. While shame can serve a purpose in alerting us to where we may have hurt another person, acted from bias, or didn't see our impact, shame's role in our culture is to keep us compliant and uphold the status quo. Knowing how shame moves through you can be helpful. Sometimes we know it's there; sometimes it's so habitual, it is running a script that we respond to without questioning—we just believe. We hope this book is helping you begin to notice and question the bullshit that happens out and inside of you. Often our most shame-supporting critical voice is aiming to protect us by keeping us small (pun not intended), scared, compliant, and flying under the radar.

Shame works because it so often speaks the voice of the dominant culture and those who have had the most power in your life. Shame is on the side of control, compliance, and being afraid. Shame backs up the parts of you that believe you have everyone fooled, that you are defective, broken, and false. That you are not worth the effort. We talked about the shame shitstorm in chapter 3, "Your Coping Is Rooted in Wisdom." The descent into painful shame reinforces concerns that we are monsters.

Shame is not motivational, either. It can create short bursts of reconciliatory-type behavior that is intended to improve optics by making decisions that look better to either the folks outside of you or the critics housed inside of you. Shame does not create sustained change. In fact, it is like rooting change in quicksand, with no foundation beneath you to keep you from sinking. In our efforts to change the world together, shame, guilt, and shunning don't create meaningful change, though they may be cathartic for those who carry harm and hurt. As Desiree Adaway reminds us, meaningful work and change is grounded in right relationship, connection, and accountability. In parallel, how can your healing be grounded in moving you toward your humanity? Can you see how ending the hustle is the work of deeper connection and accountability as you move into a relationship with yourself that you want to be in?

Shame is insidious because we don't always recognize it for what it is. What does shame feel like when it courses through you? How do you know when shame is present? Some people mistake shame for intense anxiety. It is often a hot, really yucky rising sensation that might make you feel nauseated or want to hide, bolt, disappear. It tends to create a flood of fear and self-hate, panic, and, for many, a sinking into a trauma or an acute stress response. It is not subtle, though so many people live with chronic shame it may feel usual and what their nervous systems are accustomed to.

One of the overarching constructs that operates via shame is perfectionism. Beginning to find and recognize perfectionism is a path to more freedom. We know perfectionism is a much discussed topic in circles of high profile change-makers who appear to have not truly divested from it, especially when it comes to body shame. We also know perfectionism is a piece of what upholds dominance in our culture, institutions, and relationships. Here are some questions that can root out perfectionism:

* Can you appreciate what is?

* Can you experience sufficiency versus always measuring what is inadequate?

* Do you give yourself credit? Or always assume good moments are a fluke?

* Do you make all decisions based on a diminished image of who you are to others?

* Do you talk shit about your body or other people's bodies, while making plans to "do better" with your body?

* Are you allowed to make mistakes?

Or are you always up against some idealized version of yourself that doesn't truly exist and, frankly, shouldn't? If you are focused on an idealized version of yourself, how much of your real self do you know and trust? How much are you willing to allow imperfection in the ones you love, work with, create with, and coexist with? Do you expect completeness from people's ideas, language, and efforts to value them? Is the inadequacy of your efforts or others' efforts always present in your mind? Or always conflated with who you are? Ask yourself:

* Is my body the problem or am I hurting?

* Am I a problem or is this an old story surfacing?

* Am I a problem or am I surviving, wisely coping, living my precious and necessary life?

Perfectionism is a protective flex when we can't tolerate our own humanity and we live in dehumanizing systems. And shame, in its varied somatic and cognitive forms within us, repeatedly rings the alarm bells to hustle, as Brené Brown says, for our worthiness. Perfectionism and shame keep us from doing the real work of relationship: showing up, staying humble, working through relational ruptures and harms, and letting our humanity lead.

"Who has asked you to be perfect?" was a question we pondered in a retreat we attended together a couple of years ago. The presenter, Jessica Fish, asked us to make a list of what we believe our idealized self ideally does. Maybe you want to pause and try this for a moment too?

Our lists grew easily from the constant chatter of criticism and fantasies of what could be:

Is organized

Is on time

Never hurts or disappoints anyone

Is financially responsible

Plans my life and sticks to the plan

Keeps an organized and clean house

Never yells

Doesn't check out, dissociate, or cope in a way that has "negative" consequences

Always knows what to say

Shows up for all the things and for everyone

Always helps others when I can

Journals or writes every day

Replies to all emails in a timely manner

Starts every day with a grounding practice

Doesn't spend too much time on social media

Loves to be active and move

Doesn't eat emotionally

Cooks more meals at home

Nourishes myself in a balanced and consistent way

Loves my body

Actualizing our idealized self is often dehumanizing and disembodying. "It's a way we enact self-harm," says Jessica, "and outsource ourselves for others' judgment." We do not need more plans; we need relationship with our ever-evolving humanity. You are not defective or broken, but we do know living in this world has led to these beliefs. We instead can learn how shame moves through us. And the ways it impacts how we engage with the world.

Body Trust is a reminder that you came here whole and your presence here is welcome simply because you breathe. One participant said, "Among many things, Body Trust means freedom from the prisons of had to be, must be, should be, only can be good enough if . . . Body Trust is freedom from conditional worthiness." The idealized self that shame and perfectionism fantasize about and hustle for are a product of living in a system that relies on your diminished self to profit and maintain a hierarchy of value to people based on difference. It is time to ask yourself if the values you are upholding in the pursuit of your idealized self and body are truly yours. Is there room for you in this valuation? Does your whole being, the good, the bad, the ugly, and the indifferent, have room to truly be here within The Hustle? Body Trust work asks you to reveal all of the real you.

Don't hold back. You are valid, worthy, and enough, even if you don't believe it. This is so simply because you breathe. Period.

This is a short journey. You are needed and wanted here.

MEG'S BODY STORY

In 1998, I was walking toward the Berkeley Public Library, scowling, woebegone, in a decided funk, when suddenly: rays of sunlight sparkled around me. Everything smelled like pine and cedar. My body felt warm, fluid, mobile. I noticed other people around me and was glad. There was rightness. What was actually happening is that I, several months pregnant, very tangibly experienced a hormone shift that is a hallmark of the second trimester, away from the true misery of those first three months and into sweetness, selfhood. I can still recall how surprising that moment was, what a fucking relief; like I hadn't actually breathed in a hundred days, like I couldn't see anything outside of my own struggling self.

In 2016, I was training for a 100-mile trail race. I was always nursing an injury—piriformis syndrome, bursitis of the hip, peroneal tendonitis, bone fractures. I could barely keep food down, I wasn't sleeping, and I still ran, still raced, still climbed, still cross-trained. I was "eating to compete," which meant my eating disorder was fully awake and in charge, delighted to be given such a tantalizing array of duties: restriction, denial, data gymnastics, ego maintenance, isolation, obsession, perfectionism. She felt omnipotent, miraculous. She gave me the outward appearance of what we think of in this country as "healthy." In this prized and breaking body one sunny June morning, I was summiting Mount Baden-Powell and my calf muscle ripped away from the bone. I stopped and watched as my leg created a map of bruises and blood pools and it was beautiful, a watercolor being painted. Like the walk in Berkeley, right then, something shifted, a big thing, a respect thing. It wasn't as clear, and I didn't have any answers, but I knew it was time. My friend Danny caught up to me as I stood there in the middle of the trail. "What's up?" he asked. "I can't do this anymore," I said.

By 2018, I had eaten sandwiches, pancakes, sweet potato pie, and creamed corn. Not that it was easy; there were tears and back-slides, but with the help of a good and righteous team of helpers, I was determined. I hiked with friends occasionally and walked my dog. I read short stories and drank wine. I watched food documentaries and bought new jeans. I started ovulating again, and bleeding. Then one day, in my kitchen, I felt sex come back. That dropping, full-bodied salaciousness, the definition of my queerness before ED took over. In the weeks that followed, my winking, smirking, flirtatious butch dyke tiptoed out of hibernation and reclaimed her space inside of a self that now allowed embodiment. Like the walk in Berkeley, this reminder, that my body's actions and reactions are what makes me alive, in space, in time, in physical desire, in love. That there are formidable universal truths that are housed in us, worth a listen; that we are changelings and works in progress, and that Mary Oliver's "one wild and precious life"[1] might mean fucking in a clawfoot bathtub and eating short ribs with your fingers, directly from the pot.

Part III

The Reclamation

Body Trust is a birthright, and reclamation is the process of reasserting your right to live in your body without apology, without explanation. Doing this in a world committed to body hierarchies can feel audacious. When we bravely turn our back on diet culture, many feel like they are swimming upstream when almost everybody else is going with the flow. Body Trust is a reclamation of your voice, your story, and your own damn self. In the final section of the book, we explore the nature of reconnecting with your body, discuss the phases people go through on the path to body trust, and offer practices to help deepen your roots in body trust. Our hope is that this section will help you move toward a new way of occupying, relating to, and ultimately trusting your body.

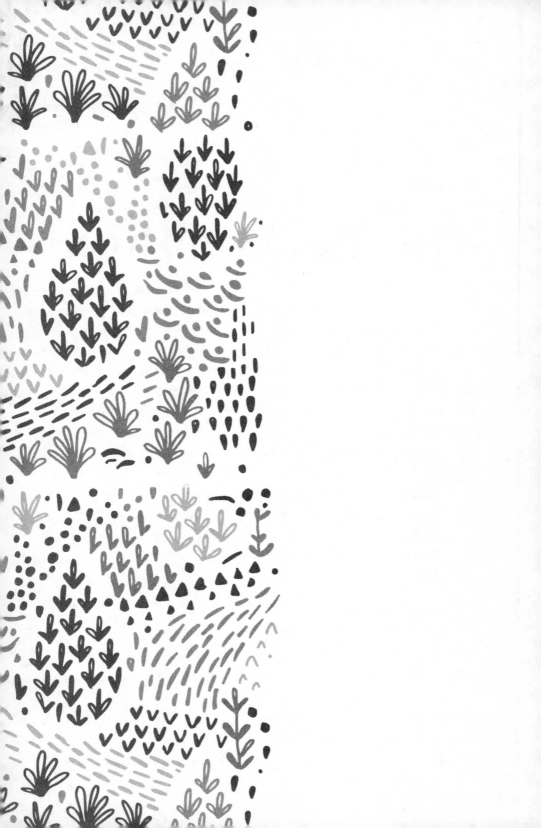

CHAPTER 8

Entering the Wilderness

Re-occupying the body is a political act.

—DR. JENNIFER MULLAN

Many, if not most, human beings engage with the world like "floating heads," cut off from the wisdom of their own embodied experience. When we disconnect from the body, we disconnect from the present moment and miss out on all kinds of information about ourselves, our bodies, our lives, our truth, and the world. We become less aware of our needs and boundaries and distanced from our gut feelings and intuition. We don't follow our rhythms or trust our own ways of knowing. We can succumb to groupthink (dominant culture) and ultimately become easier to control. Reverend angel Kyodo williams says "A disembodied culture is the direct outcome of white supremacy and mass oppression."

When we lose agency and access to our voice, we are more likely to uphold systems of oppression. We avoid confrontation and don't speak up when we know something isn't right. We internalize and prioritize all these rules and ideas about the right way to occupy and care for a body over trusting what our body tells us about our own needs for nourishment, pleasure, and connection.

Body Trust invites you back into a conversation with your body so you can begin to engage with the world and make decisions about food, your body, and your life from a more connected place. When you start to experience your body below the neck, it is a lot like entering the wilderness. You are leaving the familiar territory handed to you by the culture—the road map full of recommendations and guidelines for inhabiting and "managing your body"—and entering uncharted wild terrain. The compass you've used to navigate food and eating is no longer useful here, but you can trust that you have ancestors that came before you who were connected to their bodies and this earth, and knew how to navigate this terrain. You may feel incredibly vulnerable, and like you are flailing about without a concrete plan. It is for this reason that Savala Nolan found it helpful to think of herself as a wilderness guide during this phase of healing. You are not yet fluent in the language spoken in the foreign land that is Body Trust. You may not fully grasp it, and others still rooted in diet culture will certainly struggle to understand or help. At times, you'll want to reach back toward old, familiar ways.

We encourage you to keep returning to this work so you do not miss out on the wild, transformative part, "the part when you push past the difficulty and enter into some raw new unexplored universe within yourself," writes Elizabeth Gilbert in her book *Big Magic*.[1] Sometimes it is the experiences and circumstances that you are avoiding or looking to rush through that are the most transformative. Moving into this phase of healing is worth it, we promise! We want you to know who you've always been and what's been waiting for you beneath the shame and the self-blame, the trauma, the internalized oppression. Who you were before language and affiliation, when you were wild . . . feral . . . free. Attuned to your own rhythms and marching to the beat of your own drum. When you heard music that made your body want to move, you swayed, bounced, and danced like nobody was watching. When you were hungry, you cried out for nourishment. When you were tired, you knew to rest. You were really clear on what you liked and didn't like. What felt good and what didn't feel good. This chapter will help you understand what it means to be embodied.

The way you experience and inhabit your body changes throughout the life span as you reckon with health issues, aging, and other factors. It varies greatly depending on your intersecting identities and your proximity to power and privilege. Body Trust is not a push for a similar experience or a certain type of experience. The point of entering the wilderness and exploring what it means to be embodied isn't so you get to a place where you *always* feel at home in, or at one with, your body, or *always* like what you see when you look in the mirror. It is about understanding how we are all embodied into social systems that hold power, and then turning toward and unraveling the internalized body loathing, shame, dominance, and oppression that have made you and your body into something needing constant improvement. Our hope is this chapter will deepen your understanding of what it means to be embodied and help you create more possibilities for positive, connected experiences with food and your body.

When we came across psychologist Niva Piran's development theory of embodiment (DTE) many years ago, it opened up a whole new world to us and the work we call Body Trust. Niva has listened to hundreds of girls and women with diverse backgrounds give chronological accounts of their body stories (she calls them "body journeys"). While her research has focused on people assigned female at birth, folks across the gender spectrum in our workshops and retreats have found value in the theory and appreciate the way she connects the quality of embodied lives to societal structures of power and privilege.

In her book *Journeys of Embodiment at the Intersection of Body and Culture*, Niva explains how experiences of embodiment range from positive embodiment, described as "positive body connection and comfort, embodied agency and passion, and attuned self-care" to negative embodiment, described as "disrupted body connection and discomfort, restricted agency and passion, and self-neglect and harm." Two other important dimensions are the experience and expression of desire versus a disrupted connection to desire; and resisting objectification: subjective immersion in the body.

We are guessing it is pretty easy to identify what it is like to be disembodied and/or recall negative experiences of embodiment. But what about positive experiences? When have you felt *positively* connected to your body? What activities allow you to get absorbed in the present moment? When do you feel most alive? What fosters a positive connection to your body? What experiences help you feel a sense of belonging in the world?

We most often hear things like spending time in nature, dancing, singing, being in water, having sex, swimming, listening to live music, and spending time with people who really see and celebrate all that you are. If you have a hard time coming up with answers to the above questions, you are not alone! That's what this chapter is for. Let's take a closer look at the five dimensions of the experiences of embodiment and talk about how they connect to body trust.

Body Connection and Comfort

Take a moment to pause right now and check in with your body. Notice the position your body is currently in as you are reading this book. Are you comfortable? Is there something you could do to make you and your body a little more comfortable? Make the reading experience a little more enjoyable? Perhaps you need to go to the bathroom, get something to eat or drink, change your clothes or grab a blanket. Make some adjustments before you continue reading. This question, about what might make this a little more comfortable, is one we are rarely asked, nor do we ask ourselves.

How often do we put up with our discomfort and put off meeting even the simplest of our needs, charging forward with what we are doing? Entering the wilderness means improving the quality of connection to your body and the degree of comfort you feel in your body. This could involve addressing chronic pain, getting some clothing that fits your body today or affirms your gender identity, and building up the capacity, over time, to safely access sensations in the body.

If the idea of increasing body connection and comfort is bringing up a lot of fear for you, practitioners who specialize in trauma, EMDR (eye movement desensitization and reprocessing therapy), and somatics can help you create the resourcing and scaffolding to tolerate more body sensations and begin to discern the difference between discomfort and danger. If you start to pay attention, you may notice how your body has created adaptations, like rocking back and forth, to self-soothe and provide comfort. There's already wisdom here to be discovered. When you feel ready, you could start by bringing awareness to the parts of your body that feel less scary, like the hands and feet. Or you could just bring your hand to your heart and notice your body breathing. Some people find that when they are activated or triggered, shifting awareness to their senses (taste, touch, smell, sight, and sound) or finding an object in their view and describing it in detail helps to calm the nervous system.

Agency (Physical, Voice)

Agency connects to food and body sovereignty and is the capacity to act independently and make your own decisions. When agency is restricted, it can look like taking up less space (shrinking) literally (via weight loss) or metaphorically by not putting yourself out there or letting your presence be known. When we asked Body Trust participants, "If you could go back and talk to your younger self about diet culture, what would you want to say?" Kim S. said, "They're trying to keep you small for their reasons, not for your benefit. Dieting will condition you to never risk taking up space—physically, emotionally, intellectually, vocally, and even metaphorically—don't buy what they're selling. The price is too high."

When you are socialized to go underground, reclaiming your voice is part of the homecoming—the ability to express yourself, advocate for your needs, set boundaries, speak up in the face of injustice, and potentially lead others on this path. Exploring the questions we offer throughout this book gives you an opportunity to connect to your voice and your own knowing. You can express what you are learning through writing, art, dance, and other creative projects, or find someone you can talk to about your experiences in an honest and forthcoming way. Become aware of the times when you shrink back and defer to other people's perspectives and opinions. Sometimes it's not safe to speak up. Other times, we just need to find the courage to share what it is that we really think and/or ask for what we need. A stronger sense of agency will help you believe in your ability to contribute, succeed, and make a difference.

Brené Brown says, "Don't shrink, don't puff, stand your sacred ground."[2] Breathe into that statement for a moment. How might you begin to hold your sacred ground? To celebrate your yeses and honor your noes? How would you spend your time differently? What would you do more of? Less of? What would it be like to anchor your experiences in agency rather than restraint?

Desires

A ruptured relationship with the body impacts permission for pleasure and the ability to truly embody our desires—to both know and respond to what we want in an attuned, caring way. Many end up in a place of disowning desire. Couples therapist Esther Perel says desire is owning the wanting, and in order to own the wanting, there needs to be a self that feels deserving of the wanting.

You deserve a chance to get out from underneath what dominant culture has taught you about desire so you can discover what it is that you really want, and experience what it feels like to truly be satisfied. A participant in our School for Unlearning said, "Embodiment is the opposite of my religious fundamentalist upbringing, being taught to not trust self—and actively work against self. I've been coming back to my self for years, it's a forever journey."

What lights you up? Who are you sexually attracted to? What do you really like to eat? No apologies or disclaimers needed. You don't need to earn it or make plans for how you will repent or make up for it. Lay down your conditioning around the pursuit of pleasure. Get to know what turns you on, what makes you feel good, and what turns you off. Allowing for pleasure and satisfaction is an important part of reclaiming body trust, so there's an entire chapter coming up to help you explore this further.

Attuned Self-Care

Attunement is something you may not think about in your everyday life. It is a way we feel, sense, or listen to what's happening in our body and can include an awareness of body sensations, feelings, nervous system states, or energy shifts.

We also attune to other beings' nervous systems and emotions. We attune for greater connection and to read beneath the surface of our interactions. We attune in an attempt to keep ourselves safe. We attune to sense into what feels true and determine what feels like a lie. We may also attune to hear parts of ourselves or sense parts of others that have been quiet or sublimated.

If you've experienced trauma, stigma, or oppression, the resulting hypervigilance that has ensued to keep you safe likely means your energy and attention has been externally oriented, and rightly so. For marginalized folks, danger and a possibility of violence are part of everyday life. We aren't suggesting that you totally drop the armor. The question is, how might you begin to attend to your inner world as much as the one happening outside of you?

Many of the things people do in the name of controlling food and the body have only further disrupted attunement and contributed to patterns of self-neglect and harm. Much of what we are taught about living in a body is focused on doing things *to and on* the body as opposed to *for and with* the body. You do not need to overcome your body, nor do you have to dominate it. Body Trust is an invitation to move away from this adversarial relationship with your body toward a model of compassionate, weight-neutral self-care. "What's that?" you might be thinking. It's self-care for the sake of self-care, not to attain weight loss or impossible beauty/body standards. From a Body Trust perspective, attuned self-care means including your body and your own ways of knowing in the conversation about what kind of care makes you feel your best, and then trusting your body to sort out the weight.

Resisting Objectification—Subjective Immersion

Imagine you are on a bicycle, riding around town feeling incredibly strong and powerful. Then you pass by a storefront and catch a glimpse of your body in the reflection of the window. All of a sudden you are aware of what you look like riding the bike, and a barrage of negativity comes flooding in, tainting your experience. Your attention shifts from being absorbed in the positive experience of what it feels like riding the bike (subjective immersion) to being preoccupied with the shame and judgment of what you look like riding the bike (objectification).

We are conditioned, over time, to objectify our body (hello, body checking behaviors), and as a result, we miss out on subjective experiences that would help us to get to know ourselves, our bodies, as well as what we desire, what feels good and works for us. Niva Piran describes subjective immersion as "expressions of protest, resistance and defiance toward 'normative' pressures to adopt an external gaze and alter it [the body] to abide by appearance or other objectifying expectations."[3] Body Trust participant Maya G. shared this with us:

> *Yesterday was blazing hot. I was sweaty and needed refreshing after working on my farm for hours. I went to the local swimming hole for a bit. When I arrived, there were a handful of people there, including one of my neighbors. I took off my cover-up and walked into the water. I swam and cooled off, and when I was done, I walked up the beach to get my towel. It was one of the first summers in years that I wasn't self-conscious about my body in a swimsuit. My body is no smaller than it was last summer, or the summer before. But when I considered my body through the eyes of my neighbor and the others there, all I saw was a body that happened to be larger than some of the other bodies there. There was no shame or judgment. Just a body in a swimsuit.*
>
> *I used to think that I needed to lose weight to be comfortable in a swimsuit. What I realize now is that I was thinking about how to make other people comfortable with my body in a swimsuit. I'm not interested in making other people comfortable with my body. *I'M* comfortable with my body, and that's really the only thing that matters.*

Objectification gets in the way of people doing all kinds of life-enhancing activities, including having great sex. Many of the people we work with spend more time thinking about what their body looks like while they are having sex instead of being subjectively immersed in the giving and receiving of pleasure. We want you to feel more empowered in the bedroom and to explore what makes you feel good as opposed to what makes your body look good. There's a whole new world waiting to open up for you and your partners.

Perhaps you are already beginning to envision new possibilities for becoming more comfortable in your body and engaging with the world with embodied agency, a connection to your desires, and attuned self-care practices. We think reading fat activist and educator Shilo George's body story could help:

> As someone who has used disassociation as a trauma response for most of my life, primarily living in my head or above myself, the thing that's most helped me come back to my body is joyful movement.
>
> I've worked with a couple of different fat-positive trainers to explore movement in different ways because it's nice to have someone on your journey with you. It's also helped me feel safer exploring movement and what I really love. After a couple of months of working with a trainer fairly regularly, I noticed I have a really high pain threshold and I have my entire life. I can take a lot of pain because I know how to disassociate. I know how to extract myself from those feelings.
>
> As I've done more and more movement, I feel pain a lot more intensely than I ever have before, which is annoying in some ways. Dissociation has its benefits when I get triggered and activated with trauma, let's be real.
>
> I've recently taken up lap swimming. I had no idea I would love it as much as I do. My body really loves it. For me, being in the water is like being caressed and held and loved by the water. As a fat person and someone who doesn't have a partner, I'm often skin starving. The water is touching and cradling me in such beautiful ways. It's insular. It's just me and the water and my body. I'll be lap swimming and my brain will be like, "I'm so tired. We should stop. This is the worst thing?" Then I check in with my body, and my body's like, "This feels great. I love this. I can keep going for twenty

more laps." So I tell my brain, "Shhh. Just be quiet and take a nap, then."

Our minds are really easily manipulated, by ourselves, other people, and things like advertising. But I feel like my body—my my heart in particular—is where the truth comes from. Those parts can't really be manipulated. So what does my body actually sound like? How do I actually know I'm talking to my body and not my brain?

My body's like, "Are you sure you're talking to me right now? Because you never talked to me." And I'm like, "Can I trust you? I've been taught to not trust you and not listen to you. That you are wild and out of control. And you don't have value." I'm relearning that relationship between me and my body. Movement is one way I've started to learn to come back to myself.

Shilo's story offers insight into what entering the wilderness looks like, and how someone might increase awareness of the body, strengthen body connection, and develop somatic literacy. Somatic literacy goes beyond simply being aware of and connected to body sensations, signals, and emotional states to include discernment: the ability to catch our various reactions to stimuli, investigate them, and move into new alternatives.[4]

If you are someone who let go of the diet mentality a while ago, you may find yourself taking on the *fuck you, fuck diet culture, fuck everybody* mentality. This can look like dining out with your mother, perhaps your "chief weight stigmatizer" (a term coined by Body Trust Coach Shelby Gordon), noticing that the smoked salmon salad sounds really good for dinner but not wanting to order it because you don't want to give mom the satisfaction of thinking you made the "better choice," so you order something you don't want just to piss her off. This kind of resistance—a choice rooted in protection and opposition versus embodiment—is a necessary phase of healing. And we've noticed how some people stay there, perhaps because the trauma of deprivation was so intense. We need time to heal from depriving thoughts and behaviors before there's room for discernment. Exploring the wilderness will help you sink your roots more deeply into body trust. This involves taking risks and working the edges of your comfort zone so you can experiment with and practice the concepts we offer here. The ideas below are just that—an offering—so listen to your yeses. Honor your noes. Get curious about your resistance. And know that it is okay to say *not now* to some of this, too! This is your body. It's yours to reclaim. We trust you with your process.

Spend time in nature. You are part of this earth and the diverse array of beings that inhabit it. You belong here. You, too, are made of stardust. We wonder, What would it be like to start to see your body as part of the natural world? Shoog McDaniel, a Florida-based photographer whose work "highlights bodies and lives that are often overlooked by popular society,"[5] says, "Train your brain to see textures, shadows and rolls of your shape and how they are in deep conversation with the textures and shadows and rolls of the natural world. Bodies like oceans, bodies like boulders, bodies like sand dunes and foothills and mountains."[6] The more time we spend in nature, the more we see just how interconnected we are. A hike in the woods, watching the ocean or listening to the waves, swimming in a lake, noticing the flowers in bloom, taking in an amazing view from a vista, or removing your shoes to let your feet be in direct contact with the earth are just some of the experiences that can help us get out of our heads and back into our bodies.

Reduce body checking behaviors. When you scrutinize your body, obsessively monitor your weight, check for "flaws" in the mirror, or compare your body to others, you are essentially objectifying yourself. This kind of preoccupation with the body does not foster body connection and comfort. Our friend and colleague Rachel Cole says, "The scale takes you away from yourself. Giving it up brings you home." Keep shifting your energy and attention away from the hypervigilance.

Get reacquainted with your body through gentle touch. If you don't relate to constant scrutiny and habitual body monitoring, you might be in the camp of body avoidance, never looking at yourself or touching yourself, even when bathing. Most of us could benefit from some loving touch to increase connection to the body. You could try to do a self-massage: start with your neck, then move to your shoulders and down the arms one at a time. Or using your hands, lightly brush your arms and legs in a downward motion. Gradually increase exposure to your body over time.

Here's a practice: Place your hands over your heart, close your eyes or soften your gaze. Now take three breaths and bow your critical mind toward your compassionate heart. If this feels good, stay for a few more breaths. Notice how you feel.

Start a body gratitude practice. As we said in chapter 4, "Divesting from Diet Culture," one of the best ways to start to shift toward a more compassionate relationship with your body is by noticing how your body shows up for you every day, regardless of how you treat it. Your heart has kept beating just for you. At the end of the day, take time to reflect on and identify a few ways your body showed up and supported you.

> *My body is such a hardworking, wise, and resilient living being. She has worked so hard and endured such pain and suffering and yet she keeps showing up and fighting for my survival every day.*
>
> —LINDA T., Body Trust participant

Wear comfortable clothing. If your pants are too tight, your clothes are not comfortable, or you wear things that do not express your gender identity or who you really are, you are much more likely to have a negative experience of your body. You do not need to purchase an entire wardrobe, but if you have the money to do so, getting just a few items that feel good on you now can make a drastic difference in how you feel in your body. We recognize it may be difficult to find the right clothing since most fashion brands are not size inclusive or gender expansive. Check out our website for more ideas.

Explore gentle forms of movement. Moving the body can help foster attunement. Bring your awareness to your hands and move them around, circling at the wrists or alternating between fists and open palms. Notice sensations that arise or temperature changes. Go for a leisurely walk or change your environment and see if you can sense energy shifting or moving in your body. Put your favorite song on and dance. Close your eyes if you need to, put your hand on your heart, and just let your body sway to the music. Take a gentle yoga class with a fat positive yoga teacher. Try Tai Chi or Qigong. Check out Joyn or the Jabbie app.

Return to ritual and routine. There are simple things that are always here to help you return to yourself that you can choose to call ritual and routine. Lighting a candle. Taking a deep breath at stoplights or while waiting for transportation. Returning to your favorite quote, phrase, or poem. Listening to that song that brings you home. Putting your body in a position that signals comfort or relaxation. Uttering a few words. Checking in with a beloved person. Petting an animal. Staring at the sky.

Seek gender affirming care. If you are experiencing gender dysphoria, defined as "discomfort or distress related to incongruence between a person's gender identity and the sex assigned at birth" (*Diagnostic and Statistical Manual of Mental Disorders*, or DSM-5), you deserve access to gender affirming health care. Research shows gender confirming medical interventions (surgeries, hormones, hair removal, etc.) improve body satisfaction and reduce eating disorder behaviors. Body Trust Provider Sand Chang says, "Gender affirming health care is not cosmetic. It is life saving and life affirming care. There is no room for the 'C' word (cosmetic) in trans health."[7] Our website has resources for the trans community, and we encourage you to return to the letter to trans and nonbinary people that Sand Chang contributed for this book in chapter 2.

Consider working with a hunger scale. Reconnecting to your internal cues of hunger and fullness is one way to begin experiencing your body below the neck. Body Trust encourages you to rely less on information like nutrition, calories, points, and other calculations you may do to determine your food choices and rely more on your hunger cues and appetite. It means letting go of external messages like "It's dinnertime," "Clean your plate," or "It's bad to eat after seven p.m.," and inviting your body back into the conversation to see what works best for you and your unique life. There are a variety of hunger scales available or you can create your own. One way to do this is to draw a line down the middle of a piece of paper (we recommend using a pencil so you can edit and refine over time) and put the number 0 (zero) on one end of the line to indicate the most extreme level of hunger and 10 on the other end to signify a stuffed or uncomfortable level of fullness. And then you can fill in the line with the numbers 1 through 9. Over time, add descriptions of what mild levels of hunger feel like to you (3 or

4 on the scale) and what more ravenous cues of hunger feel like at a 1 or 2. Five is a neutral feeling where you aren't hungry or full. What might a mild level of fullness feel like to you? What does satisfaction feel like in your body? What number would you give it? Most pick a 7 or 8 out of 10. How do you know when your body is FULL, where if you keep eating, you'll start to push into pain and discomfort? We have a short video on our webpage for readers that will tell you more about using a hunger scale.

Get support. Massage therapy, cranial sacral work, somatic movement therapy, and EMDR for trauma are all modalities that can assist you in rebuilding connection with your body. If you have insurance, check to see what your benefits cover. Ask providers about sliding scale rates or equity pricing, as some have funds set aside to help cover the cost of therapy for marginalized communities. It's okay to ask to meet with a provider for a brief convo to see if they are a good fit. Be specific about what you are looking for (weight inclusive, trauma informed, trans affirming) and what accommodations your body needs. It will help you feel a little less vulnerable for your first appointment.

Explore your body story. You can use any form of artistic expression to do this: write, paint, draw, sing, dance, or use your grief altar . . . it's all a portal into knowing ourselves and honoring our process. Something especially powerful happens when we speak our truth and share our story with people who support our liberation. Even if it is just one trusted person, there is power in being witnessed.

Write letters. Another way to connect with your voice is to write letters to companies letting them know how their product(s) or business practices are impacting you and/or marginalized people in your community. Ask the companies to do better. There's no shortage of work here. We could write a letter every damn day. Also let companies that are helpful and supportive know that you see their efforts and thank them for their advocacy work.

Ask for accommodations. This one can be so hard for folks who struggle to take up space and ask for what they need. In a way, you are saying, "I'm here. My needs matter." You and your body deserve to be comfortable. Until the world is more accommodating to all bodies (write those letters!), we encourage you to make calls in advance to talk with someone about your needs, or ask a friend, loved one, or provider to help research this or consider this when making future plans. Some businesses are starting to describe their spaces with accessibility statements on their websites, letting people know about stairs/elevators, seating, parking, etc. Call restaurants to ask for details about their seating (you can sometimes find pictures on websites)—request a specific table be reserved for you. Have a concert or sporting event you want to attend? Reach out to ticket sales or customer service to find out what kind of arrangements can be made.

The process of coming home to your body, accessing what's below the neck, and returning to the innate wisdom of your own embodied experience will vary depending on your body story, your social location, and how much resourcing and support is available. Our beloved friend and colleague Carmen Cool says, "Healing is not about going away and learning to be like everyone else. Not every recovery path is right for everyone. In this healing journey, we can recapture, retrieve, and restore our ability to let our own experience of what we need surface and take the lead. It's not about never moving from some place of 'recovered'—it's about knowing how to call ourselves home."

It's unlikely that there will be a moment where you think, "Okay! I'm completely ready to descend into the wilderness!" The ability to move through your resistance and keep showing up to this work to increase access to your inner world is where healing happens. You're not gonna explore this all in one fell swoop. Over time, you'll have more discernment and feel more secure in your own knowing. You may wander away for more familiar territory and then return to the wilderness when you want to be reminded of who you really are.

Gradually, bit by bit, experience by experience, you will come home to your wild self. With time and healing, you will begin to have moments and days where you feel more neutral about your body or you aren't thinking about it much—it just is—and moments when you have more positive experiences of embodiment. The point isn't full on embodiment, 100 percent of the time. It's about allowing yourself to be fully human.

She Majestic Tree

by Angela Braxton-Johnson

Experience this beautifully majestic tree

She Majestic Tree
Big and brown
Surrounded with strength

Her hard-outer shell of lines and cracks
Allows the wild to rest on her back

She Majestic Tree's
Personal pronouns are
She, her, hers and me

Gorgeous right?!

We met on a hike
Me, on a journey home to myself
She Majestic Tree
Already there

Labored, heavy laden, misinformed and weary
From her highest peak
She could clearly see me
Down
Lurking between her toes

She treated my eyes to her fabulous treeness

Grounded
She Majestic Tree
Spreads her deep roots
Penetrating through soil, rocks and moisture

Like a tightly clenched hand
She Majestic Tree
Holds the earth that's holding her

She supports my temple
Forbidding the earth to cave beneath me

"I've got you," she says

She Majestic Tree
With arms stretched wide
Receives me
Holds me

Though miles away
She is right here

Her arms reach up to be warmed by the sun
While clouds cry tears for moisture and protection

She Majestic Tree
Supports my bountiful and weak frame
Her bigness puts my size in check
She whispers
"Aww . . . ain't you cute, with yo' lil' self!"

She offered herself as support
"Lean on me," she said
"I am here for you."

I was like an infant compared to her
Hot and thirsty from movement

I reverently, ever so gently
Placed my hand on her ankle
I leaned in
Shifting part of my weight onto her
She Majestic Tree didn't budge

"I don't want to hurt you,"
I said to her
"I've been told I'm too fat,
Too big, too much, too . . ."

She interrupted my nonsense by waving her branches
I was not too much for her

Oblivious of me
She danced with the wind
Together they provided a breeze of refreshment
Quieting my false and toxic thoughts

With gratitude, praise and a newfound contentment
I got down on my knees
Rested on her toes
And thanked God Almighty for this beautiful creation

She, like me
Was wonderfully made

Takings sips from my thermos I drank in her greatness
Basking in her shade

She released a few leaves onto my head
Crowning me with her glorious essence

Surrendered to rest
I hugged her hard and scratchy ankles
Allowing all of me to rest on her strength

She lovingly laughed
And said, "That tickles."[8]

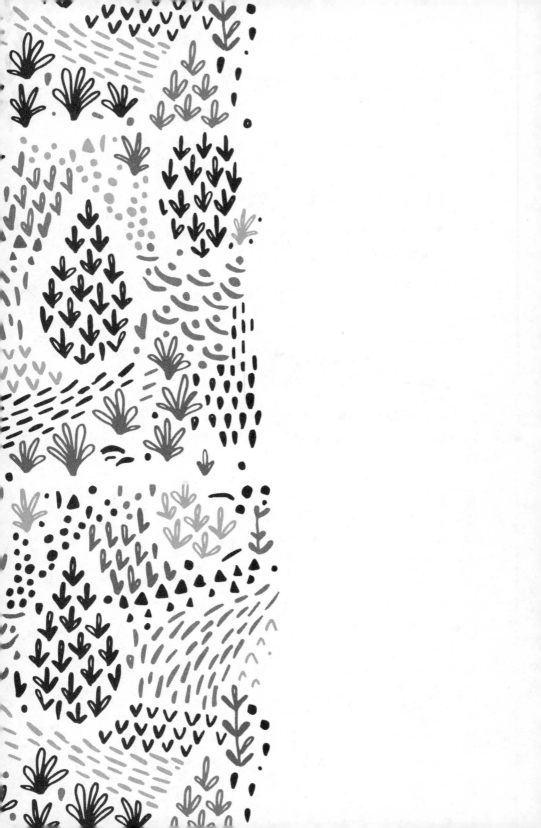

CHAPTER 9

Allowing for Pleasure and Satisfaction

I touch my own skin, and it tells me that before there was any

harm, there was miracle.[1]

—adrienne maree brown,
Pleasure Activism: The Politics of Feeling Good

ody Trust is a reclamation. Of knowing. Of wanting. Of listening. Of pleasure. Body Trust work is a process of reclaiming our bodies after internalizing diet culture and oppressive ideals about our bodies, which further distances us from ourselves as we hustle for the perfect body. When all this happens, we become numb and often lose access to many embodied experiences, including emotions, pleasure, and satisfaction.

"Body Trust means having a deep connection with my own body as a part of myself, rather than a separate entity," says Body Trust participant Leanne W. "It means being able to feel the physical sensations of hunger, fullness, satiety, and the full range of physical expressions of emotions and being able to trust that those sensations are my body's way of communicating with my conscious mind. Being able to respond to these sensations with nonjudgmental and wise actions that nurture and support me."

In the last chapter, we explored the five dimensions of the experiences of embodiment that emerged from Niva Piran's research, one of which is the experience and expression of desire. Many factors throughout the life span impact embodiment and thus access to pleasure, and a complicated relationship with food and the body often includes a disrupted relationship with desire. Reclaiming pleasure is an act of resistance in a culture that has made indulgence a "dirty word." We hope Body Trust work supports an awakening of sensation, emotion, and joy. Your sensations and emotions were not to blame for the harm or intensity you may have experienced in your life, but they were often too much to feel to survive and keep going.

The culture has deemed expression of desire and pleasure suspect in women, poor people, Black people, trans people, Native folks, disabled people, and every other marginalized identity that exists. When our sense of self has been challenged and disenfranchised, we have to find the path that brings us back to our very right to want, express, and ask for pleasure. Desire, pleasure, and joy take up space and say, "I'm here." It is not a shrinking back, but rather an expansion and expression of ourselves. We believe that pleasure, in the absence of shame and guilt, is a healing force. Many of us have a "restricting" or "depriving" voice that works hard to limit or silence our wanting. Rediscovering, embodying, and allowing for pleasure is an important part of reclaiming body trust. When we are able to listen to and view our own longing as valuable, we can begin to meet our own needs respectfully.

Our loss of pleasure has roots. Artist Elwing Su'o'ng Gonzalez asks:

> *Whom have you been raised to please? How has your existence been tailored to please? What are the ways we are taught to put parts of ourselves, our desires, our opinions, our feelings, our identities on the back burner in the interest of someone*

or something else, at the great expense of shrinking or losing ourselves? How much of your self-development has been done to please/not be excluded by/be validated by/not provide the ridicule of them or them or them or them and do they reciprocate the respect and concern? We must play roles to survive but: Do you remember what you really want and feel and who you really are? Do you deeply change or deny yourself to be desirable to people, to make a "good wife," to get your family's approval, to be accepted by people of a higher economic class, to feel you belong in the mainstream, to feel like you deserve to be at your college/job/neighborhood? Do you really want to do the things you do?

Pleasure is a necessary, core intelligence of humanity. It is essential in relationships, self-care, part of our basic needs, and it has a role in what we create, innovate, and how we change our world and evolve. Pleasure has the potential to be woven through all aspects of our being and how we show up. So it matters when it has been made suspect, secondary, or shameful.

What did you learn about pleasure growing up? Who did you learn it from?

Erica G. shared this story with us:

I love watching home movies of my childhood. In most ways I had an extremely loving and warm family life, and I love to watch that dynamic in play. My mom filmed everything, including my first birthday. My parents put a huge birthday cake in front of me and pointed the video camera. They started asking me questions as I dove in hands and then face first. Everyone was oohing and awwwwing at how cute it was, and laughing at my vigor and excitement around the cake. I had never had sugar before. In the midst of all of the attention, you can hear my mom off camera say, "Five pounds, honey." I was one year old. I had barely started living and I was being indoctrinated into fat phobia and food and weight gain anxiety. It's so sad. I have come a long way with my parents on the subject of food and body shame. They have fully consented to my sharing this story. We all hope other children don't have to fear food and go through the emotional and physical pain I went through to achieve even a base level of body trust.

Consider your gut reaction when you hear the word "pleasure." What have you learned to believe about people who seek pleasure? Are they trustworthy and reliable? Can they be leaders you trust? Perhaps since you have started reading this book, you have begun to consider or have actually played with the possibility of guilt-free eating. Perhaps you have wanted to have that experience, but have not figured out how to let go afterward. Some of you may be coming at this from a lot of years of "fuck you" eating, and are wondering if that has been pleasurable. For some, it really is. For others, it's fraught with disconnection and self-judgment.

One of the ways we begin to consider pleasure in our relationship with food is to notice the difference between being full and feeling satisfied. Fullness is pretty basic, like the sense that there is enough food in your stomach, that you are no longer hungry, that it might be a while before you get hungry. Satisfaction is a far more full-bodied, emotional reaction. Satisfaction says, "Damn, that was good." Or, "No one makes spaghetti like my grandmother—the best!" You can be satisfied but not necessarily full, like after an amazing ice cream cone or the perfect peach.

What do you think of when you hear the words "appetite" and "hunger"? How are they different? Hunger signals a need; appetite connects to desire. Hunger says, "I need food." Appetite says, "What do I want? What sounds good?" Let's take a closer look: Andi goes to lunch with a coworker and they want to get the fried chicken sandwich but they fear being judged for this choice (there's a lot of diet talk at the office), so they order the grilled chicken salad. The salad tastes okay and provides enough food for them to feel full, but they're left wanting something else after lunch because they don't feel satisfied. If they'd had had what they really wanted for lunch on this particular day—the fried chicken sandwich—they might have walked away from the meal feeling really satisfied and done with food for a while. Satisfaction is a relative of pleasure—perhaps a gateway—and is often missing from the lives of people who have disordered relationships with food and their body. We must stop marketing the myth that food is fuel or that we are better off eating like cavepeople. The toxic masculinity and whiteness that informs nutrition restraint is infuriating: no feelings, follow the rules, you can't be trusted, intuition and desire are dangerous ways of knowing compared to science and numbers. Bullshit. Restriction and restraint have come to be central to the mainstream white-woman ideal. It fills our social media feeds; the performance is measured and minimal with restrained appetite and emotion. However, control is an illusion. We are humans and our relationship with food is complex and involves our hearts, our history, our brains, our hands, our memories, and our desires.

We wonder, when was the last time you felt truly satisfied after a snack or meal? Do you remember what you ate? Where you were? Who you were with? And what made that bit of pleasure possible? Maybe it was just damn good food? Or maybe there was more to it, like you were in a pleasant atmosphere with loved ones who make your heart swell. Or maybe you felt permission to enjoy it? Or you had your hands in the process of making the food and that made it extra satisfying? What made it good?

From working with people over the years, we find folks need to lean into, explore, and feel satisfaction to help heal their relationship with food. For many people it's the secret sauce. If satisfaction has not been a valued part of eating, you may find that in order to come back into pleasure with food, you need to experience satisfaction once a day or more. Our relationship with food improves when it happens regularly.

One topic that needs some unpacking is the way we talk about and label "emotional eating." There are some common patterns that live under the surface of our awareness related to what we call emotional eating. If you "try to be good" by restricting or restraining food most of the day, you will likely reach for more food in the evening. We understand why folks call this emotional eating or even bingeing, but we aren't sure that's always an accurate description. We do believe that at the end of a long day you are feeling more emotional, especially if you haven't had enough to eat. We also appreciate that our bodies are smart enough to turn our attention toward food when we aren't eating enough—and that can be through hunger, unrelenting thoughts of food, cravings, etc. Those times when you can't get dinner on the table without eating everything first, and then you eat dinner and snack more afterward, may very well be your body's reach for homeostasis—to bring your body back into balance by getting enough food to meet your needs. This is not purely the stuffing of emotion that we attribute the eating to. We also know that in this part of The Cycle, you may be feeling a lot when this happens, including anxious, frustrated, disgusted, sad, and worried. You still need to get enough to eat. And if you have dieted, restricted, and restrained your eating throughout your life, we guess that what you believe is enough food might not be enough for your body.

Some questions worth asking: When was the last time you experienced guilt-free pleasure when eating? And what about in general? What made it pleasurable? Did you need others to help? Did you make space to enjoy? What happened and why? Sometimes we can create these experiences for ourselves but are unable to share them with others because it would not be understood or condoned. Maybe in your queer community it's okay but not among your work friends. Maybe your family has history with pleasure and joy, but your partner does not. Maybe pleasure was okay or natural for some in your life but there was a different set of rules for others. It may help to take a step back and think about who in your family, in the culture, is allowed to experience pleasure. Whose desire was centered in your household growing up? Whose comfort was prioritized? Who catered to those desires through unpaid labor?

When we bring these questions to workshops and retreats, the answers are important but unsurprising. Most people say the men in the family had the most access and permission to seek pleasure. Some say no one. Some say the children. No one has yet said the women in the family. No one has said anyone or everyone. Shena J., a Body Trust participant, shared this with us:

> *Body Trust has opened my eyes to the fact that I spent decades serving the needs of others through abusing my body to help them stay comfortable. It helped me learn that by doing this, I am harming both them and myself by instilling worth into a system that damages all of us.*
>
> *I have become incredibly angry at the underlying desire I wasted so much of my time and energy on to become thin. I could've spent my time so much more efficiently and been truly engaged in my growth as a person rather than trying to achieve thinness that would only momentarily serve onlookers.*

* Who in our culture is entitled to own their desire?

* Who gets to know what they want to eat and how much?

* Who is entitled to a sexual appetite?

* Who is trusted to spend?

* Who is trusted to lean into pleasure without having their productivity questioned?

If you had a chance to take a pleasure vacation where there were no deadlines, no timelines, no to-do lists, and no expectations or judgments of you, where your pleasure and satisfaction were centered and celebrated, what kinds of sights, sounds, textures, objects, flavors, and experiences would be there? (Shout-out to Dawn Serra for offering us this question for our Body Trust Summit.) Pleasure has often been associated with *too much* or *not enough*, and shame and guilt are measuring sticks that are often close behind. Allowing for pleasure and satisfaction is one of the more challenging parts of this work. It's not considered mandatory but extra or "if I get around to it."

Pleasure is our birthright. We are born to experience joy with the same frequency and fervor we feel pain, shame, frustration, hope, worry, and anticipation. Joy, pleasure, and satisfaction all too often hit our radar as something suspect or dangerous. An unfortunate and erroneous relationship has been established between pleasure and too much. Based on our culture's warped estimation, we are on such a slippery slope when it comes to joy and pleasure that we'd better devise some complicated equations to allow ourselves *just a little*, or skip it all together. Capitalism is warped, and probably does better if we are wanting but we think we shouldn't have.

We want you (and all of us) to have a clearer sense of why—as adrienne maree brown, author of *Pleasure Activism*, says—pleasure is a measure of our freedom. We do not believe that pleasure will make you out of control, and frankly, if it does for a while, that's what may be needed. Honestly, there is nothing more satisfying than having clear sight on how pleasure functions in your life. A place to start is back in your body story, your ever evolving body story, to remember step by step where it went missing. As we have said before, we do not come into this life fretting about food or our body. As infants we are equipped to signal to others, unapologetically, what we want and need.

There was a time for many of you that signaling what you wanted and needed became a problem for or was judged by others. Your natural developmental push and pull between independence and need, which goes on throughout childhood and adolescence, may have been cut short by competing needs in your family or with your caregivers or circumstances. Perhaps they didn't fully understand your developmental needs. Perhaps they also didn't understand their own conflicts with need and want. Perhaps they wanted to protect you from wanting because of their lifetime of disappointment. Perhaps, despite their best effort, there just wasn't enough to go around. Perhaps they felt control was safer for you. And, likely, the culture dictated what was good to your family, and your caregivers decided how to keep you safe within those constructs. Either way, ideas about wanting, needing, joy, and pleasure may have become confusing and might still be.

When we talk about pleasure we are talking about all in, go for it, no guilt, who is watching anyway, YOLO, pleasure for the sake of pleasure. We are not talking about experiencing pleasure but feeling guilty the whole time. We aren't talking about pleasure that eighteen of your nearest and dearest have sanctioned so you know it's okay. We would actually like pleasure to be so a part of your life that you feel you are enjoying life more than you have before.

We have such roots in having pleasure be punishable or sinful that we cannot envision being safe with it. Pleasure, then, has been reconfigured, bargained with, minimized, and squashed to make it okay under certain circumstances. Utter bullshit. We are designed for pleasure. You should have more freedom internally and externally to decide what to do with that. Pleasure is so deeply suspect and implicated in many "bad" things, including our relationship with food, that the general rule has been to cut it off at the knees by avoiding it, lying about it, sneaking, or feeling guilty about it. And this has messed us up a bit. There are roots we can't ignore: puritanical roots, white supremacy culture, patriarchal versions of God, control over women and other marginalized people.

It's worth pondering: Why, when people are talking about, say, a huge banana split, or a night of deeply satisfying sex, a shopping spree, or a weekend on the couch, do we feel more internal contraction and judgment than celebration from anyone but our besties? Why are so many of us apologetic? When has a cookie or even a box of cookies ever truly been a slippery slide into a danger zone? *Never in the history of humanity.* Why, when we take a day off from "something that is good for us," is there suspicion about our value or intentions? Investigate the story of how you became so suspicious of yourself. Those roots need to be exposed.

We need a cultural reckoning with the pathologizing of desire. We understand, especially through some parenting education, that stigmatizing and pathologizing desire, wanting, and longing puts a greater emphasis on the wanting. And if the desire itself is problematized, folks are more likely to internalize their badness, that something is wrong in them for having the desire. Shame is equated with the sense that "I am bad," based on Brené Brown's research, instead of "I've made a mistake or done something wrong."[2] Compulsive behavior, in some cases, may be an outcome of shame cycles when human desire is pathologized, not a sign of something being deeply wrong with an individual person. We understand you may have been deeply hurt and traumatized. This does not make you broken.

Addiction is not hedonism. That association is a true dumbing down of a layered and complex physiological and psychological experience rooted in survival and coping with systemic and institutional oppression, pain, and trauma. We are not "potential addicts" because we want sugar, sex, attention, and stuff. Do we notice our minds quickly moving to addiction, worry about financial ruin, and a general distrust of people? A lot of the rhetoric around recovery talks about admitting one's "powerlessness" over the "physical dependency" on the substance. Guilt and shame are used as motivators even if you have to "white-knuckle it." While these concepts have helped people reckon with their substance use, they are not as helpful when reproduced in diet culture. This type of categorizing of habits and ritualized behaviors actually enables the trauma and addiction industries to bypass the social determinants and stressors and zero in on behavioral interventions. As our colleague and friend Carmen Cool has said, "The goal of therapy should never be to help people adjust to oppression."[3] We can move toward frameworks that help people but also have an impact larger than individual healing. Cultural, systemic, and institutional change is what is truly needed.

Think about the lies you are here to defy (Desiree Adaway). Think about how you've been lied to about yourself. You are not a walking ticking time bomb because you want. Also, gaining weight from feeding and nourishing yourself adequately will not devastate you. You must experience fullness, satisfaction, joy, and pleasure to trust in your wholeness. As much as seeking distraction and coping with food, sex, relationships, etc., can be a way of coping, pleasure is a part of healing. One does not negate the other. The denial of pleasure and enjoyment are central to eating disorders, disordered eating, healthism, diet culture, nutritionism, ableism, and the like. Your desire is being concern-trolled and policed by those with mouthpieces, degrees, and platforms who have not reckoned with this for themselves. One way to get out from under the denial of pleasure and at least see what rises to the surface is to ask yourself: If I could do/eat/experience anything right now and be guaranteed that it wouldn't affect my health, weight, or reputation, what would I want to do?

Rachael Ringwood, a Body Trust Provider and therapist in Portland, Oregon, shared some of her story about discovering pleasure:

> *Experiencing the sensuous delight of a good latté—with that velvety foam and its art—was my submission into pleasure. I was first treated to coffee by a captivating and assertive friend, who made no apologies for their bliss. At the time, I half humorously joked that I was a victim of pleasure, because it was something that overtook me more than it was a choice. The notion that I saw myself as a pleasure victim is sad to me now that I understand and believe everybody deserves access to pleasure.*
>
> *Until my basic needs were met, I was floundering in survival mode and experienced food insecurity to the point I was eating out of garbage cans, waiting for people to be done with their food and fishing out their discarded take-out boxes. That velvety latté was extra, it was so extra. I didn't believe I de-*

served it. Before I could say yes to myself and others experiencing pleasure, I had to heal from the internalized judgment I experienced as a person of color parenting single with low income. I had to learn I was worthy of sustenance, excess, and joy. I wasn't familiar with coffee shops, and by no mistake I was drawn to a queer one. That bougie five-dollar coffee was an access point—an invitation through my senses—to experiencing something warm and communal.

When we have enough space beyond survival that we can pause and ask our body what it wants to experience, and have the ability to provide for our wants, it is vitalizing. It is also deeply privileged.

The more marginalization someone experiences, the more suspect and even criminalized their pursuit of pleasure may be. This is exemplified in the cannabis industry by the number of Black people who are behind bars for distribution and possession, while the newly legal and recreational cannabis industry is led by White folks who profit freely. Black and brown people's bodies are hypersexualized, a remnant from slavery and colonization attempts to shift blame for the sexual violence Black, Indigenous. and people of color experienced at the hands of colonizers and slave owners. We know a group of Black folks enjoying each other's company can be stupidly read as suspect or dangerous to intrusive white folks who are passing by. Psychologist Angel Dunbar speaks to some of the effects of this on Black children:

* Black children experience harsher disciplinary action at school,

* Their neutral facial expressions are viewed as more aggressive and threatening than their White peers, and

* They are more likely to be expected to misbehave even when engaging in normal play.[4]

Dunbar goes on to say, "When it seems like Black children are mistreated for expressing anger, fear, joy, or for simply existing, it can be a daunting task to figure out how to best protect them from harm while also allowing them to live and thrive unapologetically."

Joy and pleasure are necessary to humanity—essential to life—thus they are political. They should not be regulated by power, especially power that will not speak about or name itself as such. We harm others when we regulate, police, control, pathologize, and vilify joy, expression, connection, survival, pleasure, art, and community. And we harm ourselves.

Fatness is another intersection whose expression of satisfaction, joy, and pleasure is often publicly monitored, something thin people do not often experience. If you are fat, what is it like for you to seek pleasure in public? And in private? What do you have to assume others are thinking about you in order to protect yourself? Do you believe you deserve pleasure, regardless of the naysayers around you? Are you fighting a sense that you should be earning it? Fat folks do not have equal access to the pleasures that thin folks may not recognize as privileges. Can you go shopping and try on clothing in a store? Is furniture made with you in mind? When you book a flight, do you think twice because of the limitation of airline seats and the shame that others cast upon you when you share space with them? Can you go to the grocery store and buy snacks without commentary? Are you seen as a viable sexual person? Do you have to question if sexual interest in you is a fetish or simply coming from a genuinely interested and evolved enough human?

We relish in the celebration of fat bodies that can be found on social media. #FatVanity affirms the gloriousness of the fat body and attempts to show fatness through a fat gaze instead of a thin one. This idea challenges the notion that people "glorify obesity" by enjoying their fat bodies or trusting in the attractiveness of themselves despite the inaccurate and harmful idea that fat can't be attractive.

One of the challenges we are presented with as we move toward healing our relationship with food and body is that we are confronting the ways that numbing through food, compulsive exercise, and ongoing body improvement plans have numbed more than just our unwanted thoughts and feelings. It has likely numbed it all. Brené Brown writes about how we cannot selectively numb our emotions.[5] So if we are numbing sadness because it is too much to feel or deal with (because it can be sometimes), then we inadvertently also numb joy, anger, happiness, fear, etc. We numb it all. Getting curious about pleasure can mean reawakening—or discovering for the first time—the degrees of sensation and emotional feeling that have been buried for a while. One of the side effects of awakening to sensation again is awakening to pleasure. This can be great news. This can also be confronting. Opening to and owning pleasure is part of the healing journey.

Why? The erotic is an essential part of our being. The erotic can refer to our sexual self, certainly, but the erotic is about much more than sex. The erotic is essentially *the language of the body*. You may just start here:

Where do you hear yes in your body? And where do you hear no? As you read our words, what is rising in you? What is shutting down?

In an unpublished piece titled "Why Nutrition Needs the Erotic," radical dietitian Lucy Aphramor writes:

> *The erotic is the anti-thesis to body shame: with the erotic, our emotions, our fleshiness, our appetites will not be used against us. We can learn to accept and respect our bodies and sensations. We can learn to listen to our emotions and appetites and trust them as sources of information. We can stop objectifying our bodies, and others', and start to heal the mind-body disconnect taught in conventional nutrition. Including the erotic means we bring back the body and non-rational ways of knowing into the intellectual landscape: this changes everything.*

The erotic can be reclaimed and become our wisest teacher—a guide toward what we are here to express. Trauma often means shutting down aspects of yourself to keep you safe. This chilling of our bodies and our being is a part of our wise coping. Eroticism, pleasure, joy, and satisfaction are a piece of the awakening and the reclamation.

Have you ever thought about what lights you up? What gives you life? It's also important to know what dims your light or turns you off. We posed these questions in one of our online School for Unlearning sessions and participants shared the following:

WHAT GIVES ME LIFE?

Dancing

Music

Good books

Activism

Being near water

Deep conversations

Spending time with like-minded people

WHAT TURNS ME OFF?

Perfectionism

When I close myself off

Sublimating pleasure/prioritizing the pleasure of others over my own

Saying yes when I need to say no

When I stop sharing myself or my needs

Not eating enough

In her book *Mating in Captivity*, Esther Perel talks about the erotic as essential to meaningful survival. She'd been curious about her husband's work with victims of torture and had asked him how he knows when a torture victim comes back to life:

> It turns out that people come back to life when they are able to reconnect with creativity, vitality, and with the opposite of vigilance. You can't play when you're vigilant. You can't play when you're anxious. You can't play when you're fearful. You can't play when you don't trust. That's when I made the connection. There were two groups in the community of Holocaust survivors that I grew up with in Antwerp. There were the houses that just had survived, but you felt deadness in them: from the curtains being down, to the heaviness, antihedonism, and the inability to experience the pleasure of being alive. And then you had the houses of people who had really experienced eroticism as an antidote to death and knew how to keep themselves alive; to stay connected to vitality and vibrancy and exuberance and joy and force.[6]

We've witnessed this very difference in people we've worked with who are recovering from eating disorders. There are those who do not die and then there are those who come back to life, who reconnect to this quality of aliveness and vitality . . . the erotic. The Hustle, this process of self-improvement, has been deadening. Disordered eating, body distrust, body blame, racism, and sexism have been deadening. Many people trying to perfect food and their body are hoping they will move closer to feeling alive when XYZ happens. And it doesn't happen. Or it's fleeting. Or the closer you get, the more hypervigilant, anxious, fearful, and distrustful you are of yourself.

Audre Lorde, one of the most foundational teachers and writers on the erotic, said, "The erotic is a measure between the beginnings of our sense of self and the chaos of our strongest feelings. It is an internal sense of satisfaction to which, once we have experienced it, we know we can aspire."[7]

What are we reclaiming? The ability to feel, express, discern, and destigmatize wanting. Meaningful, non-performative embodiment. Hunger. Appetite. Voice. Agency. A reconnect to desire housed in and expressed from our own bodies.

Ask yourself, What scares me the most about allowing or pursuing pleasure, joy, and satisfaction? And what happens if I continue as things are? What would be different if the people in my life really, truly wanted me to enjoy my food, to know pleasure, and celebrated my desires?

In her "Power in Pleasure" course, sex and relationship coach Dawn Serra offers Three Pillars of Pleasure:[*]

1. **Pleasure happens only in the present moment, so presence is required.** You'll arrive and leave, show up and exit. A pleasure practice invites us to keep returning to ourselves and to feel more fully. This is because pleasure happens only in the body. It is an emergent experience that comes from within. In order to connect with your pleasure, you must arrive and feel what is happening now.

2. **Context and choice define each moment of every potentially pleasurable experience.** (*Safety must come first.*) Our ability to access pleasure is informed by things like the people around us, the stories we carry, the way we feel about our bodies, what has happened throughout our day, how much emotional labor or caretaking we are doing, and whether we truly feel we have a choice about what is happening to us (obligation and "should" often cut us off from our pleasure). This is why it is often easier to access pleasure when we are on vacation versus when we are at

---

[*]   Dawn would like to acknowledge the work of Betty Martin in her writing of Pillar #1 and Emily Nagoski's influence in Pillar #2.

home surrounded by laundry, bills, and to-do lists as long as our arm. Shifting the context often shifts the experience.

3. **The senses/sensory input are the gateway.** What is the taste of home? What is the smell of yes? What sounds make you smile? Though pleasure can be complicated for many of us, when we practice turning toward our senses, we begin to discover just how abundant pleasure can be in our lives. As we develop the ability to notice what feels good, we begin discerning our likes and dislikes, our longings and desires. This lays the groundwork for being able to articulate our wants and needs in genuine, body-affirming ways.

Here is a final question for you. If you woke up tomorrow and never had to worry about being maligned for a physical characteristic again, if you had access to safety and could feel into your wholeness, what would you want to do more of? What would you want to do less of? Trust your knowing.

CHAPTER 10

Reclaiming Movement

Human beings need food and movement to survive. Diet culture steals food and movement, deeply pathologizes them, then commodifies them and sells them back to us.[1]

—VIRGIE TOVAR

I f you've had a complicated relationship with food and your body, it is unlikely that somehow your relationship with movement has gone unscathed. Just the title of this chapter can bring up a lot for people and you might already notice some resistance. So we want you to know up front that you won't find any "shoulds" in here. There's no rhetoric about getting 10,000 steps or 30 minutes a day.* Or rules about what activities you need to be doing. No recommendations for how often or how long you need to do them to count. We want to give you an opportunity to think about your relationship with movement, aka exercise, fitness, or physical activity, and how it has been stolen from you,

---

* It turns out 10,000 steps a day is not an evidence-based recommendation, and yet public health institutions and health care organizations hopped on that bandwagon, handing out pedometers and encouraging people to track their steps.

co-opted by diet culture and what Ilya Parker has coined "toxic fitness culture" (more on that later). There's a lot to unpack here and this subject is not to be taken lightly. We've been deeply humbled witnessing what happens in a room when we explore people's relationship with movement over the course of their lifetime. Hint: get the tissues, maybe?

We've chosen not to use the words "exercise" or "physical activity" in Body Trust work because of how loaded they are for most people who've been stuck in chronic patterns of dieting and disordered eating. Movement is something we were born into; exercise is something we've been sold to improve our health or mold our bodies. Human beings have an innate connection to moving the body. Diet culture and the cosmetic fitness industry rob us of our agency. There's a sense that we are no longer in charge of what we know to be true about our body. That they know more than we do about our body. And when you have a marginalized identity, this "I know more about what you need" reinforces oppression.

There's so much the fitness world doesn't take into consideration because many people's bodies have been left out of the conversation. There is systemic fatphobia and ableism in almost all exercise, wellness, yoga, and fitness spaces, which makes these spaces especially unsafe for fat people, disabled people, trans people, and people with a history of disordered eating. Discussions about movement, including this chapter, will have elements of ableism because language about movement is often expressive of more able-bodied people's experiences with moving.

Movement should not be a mandate. You are not required to perform health or pursue fitness to be worthy of love, respect, and belonging. There is no moral obligation to move your body. In fact, not everyone reading this book will be able to explore movement for a whole host of reasons, including disability, chronic pain, access to supportive therapies, and more. It's not as simple as "just do it."

"Toxic fitness culture is rooted in white supremacist ideals regarding health, ability, size, gender, age and beauty," says Ilya Parker, founder of Decolonizing Fitness. "It is intertwined with diet culture, and both place blame on an individual for the ways their body shows up in this world."[2] In an article titled "How to Tell if Your Relationship with Exercise Is Toxic," Ilya gives several examples of toxic fitness culture:

* The promotion of fitness for the sole purpose of weight loss.

* Personal trainers unwilling or unable to modify exercises that support your unique body.

* The belief that you're not working hard enough if you haven't achieved thinness.

* Personal trainers who aren't registered dietitians giving diet advice.

* Personal trainers who don't believe you when you say you need to stop and who encourage you to push through pain.

* The belief that beating your body up makes for a good workout.

* The belief that your body has to get smaller or toned when you engage in fitness, and if it doesn't, then you're doing something wrong.

* Thinking diet and exercise are the only ways for someone to take care of themselves.

* Cultivating fitness spaces that aren't accessible or affirming to a diverse group of bodies.[3]

It is rare to see diverse representations of bodies in the world of fitness and athletics. When you think of a fit body or an athletic one, who comes to mind? Your first image is probably someone who fits society's narrow definition of a "good" body—a flat stomach/six-pack abs, toned arms and legs, little to no visible cellulite. We doubt most readers of this book think of a larger-bodied person or a disabled person. Until very recently, there hasn't been activewear available for fat bodies, and you didn't see any body diversity in catalogues selling activewear.

Fat bodies are rarely portrayed positively in the media, and when a story airs about a fat person running a marathon, the concern trolls swoop in with their fat shaming and accusations that the article is glorifying obesity. Fat people are constantly told to "move their fat asses," but when they do, they are harassed by strangers passing by in cars or people coming up to them in the gym saying things like "You have to start somewhere. Good for you." Accessible yoga teacher Shannon Kaneshige says, "I lost DECADES of movement due to the trauma of exercise and fear of violence."[4]

As we age, we become more and more aware of this pervasive weight stigma. Movement shifts from a way to engage with the world, connect to our bodies, and actively play with friends and family toward an aesthetic of health and a whole host of performative bullshit. Motivations to move become rooted in cosmetic fitness, i.e., "looking fit." Many if not most people working out in a gym are there to "get rid of this or that," sometimes because they believe it is what's needed to be fit or healthy. Personal trainers and fitness professionals often collude with these notions because they too have been indoctrinated into these harmful societal constructs and their training has done little to challenge their socialization. They may even struggle with their own disordered relationship with food, exercise, and their body.

Despite popular belief, the truth is fitness doesn't have a "look"; people of all weights, shapes, and sizes run marathons, practice yoga, dance, climb mountains, box, swim, and do CrossFit. You cannot look at someone and assess their health status or fitness level. Research has actually shown, time and time again, that fitness and fatness can coexist.[5]

It is no wonder many of us end up in a relationship with movement that feels more adversarial than connected, enjoyable, or playful. There's an attitude of doing things *to and on* the body as opposed to *for and with* the body. People in our programs say that before childhood play became exercise, there were fewer rules and no expectations. Movement was a choice, with more ownership and agency. We hear things like, "I wasn't focused on being good at any of these things, it just felt like freedom"; and "I never liked swim meets and the recitals—my favorite moments were the embodied moments when I was in the water or on the dance floor at the rehearsal studio, when I could just let myself be and get lost in myself." At some point, movement turns into something that we should do or are supposed to do instead of something that we want to do because we like how it makes us feel, we sleep better, it helps us manage chronic pain, we release pent-up stress and anxiety, we laugh and have fun with others, and (insert any and all nonappearance-related benefits).

We didn't think we could write a book that challenges the dominant paradigm about weight and health without including a chapter to help you divest from toxic ideas about fitness. You can explore this on your own terms and in your own time. For many people we work with, the idea of moving their body brings them face-to-face with what it has meant to live in their body—the stigma and trauma, the lack of privilege and access, the changes in physicality, fitness, ability/disability—so be gentle with yourself. The reckoning is often more confronting and emotionally charged than we expect some folks to have words for. What's happened to many of us in terms of movement requires a bending toward forgiveness to really acknowledge our body story and begin to externalize the real harm in the culture that has interrupted your relationship with your body and with movement. It shouldn't have been this way. Ultimately, we hope this chapter will help you reclaim a sense of agency with movement so you can determine what feels best for you and your unique body moving forward.

What's come between you and your relationship with movement? When and how did active play become exercise? You might start by thinking about what movement was like as a child. How active were you? What do you remember about the activities you were doing? What did you like about them? What made those activities possible? Or what got in the way of you being able to do the things you enjoyed doing as a child?

Now fast-forward to your experiences in middle school and high school. What was your activity level like then? What were you doing? What changed during these years? What opportunities were you given to explore movement? What got in the way of you accessing the kinds of activities you enjoyed doing?

When we explore these seemingly innocuous questions, we start to see how intersections of race, class, ability, gender, and fatness impact what our relationship with movement has been, as well as what it is like today. We hear about parents who weren't available for sports because they were working multiple jobs to make ends meet, neighborhoods that weren't safe to go outside and play, and towns that didn't have sports for kids with physical disabilities. Some women share how their brothers were signed up for sports but the girls in the family weren't allowed to play. Several have told us about how their passion for dancing and ice skating was hijacked by the standards of beauty in the sport. When they didn't meet a certain aesthetic, they stopped doing what they loved, sometimes because they were thrown out when their bodies no longer "fit the mold." Another shared how their parents would make them run after dinner while they drove the car alongside them because they wanted them to lose weight. And then there's the twelve-year-old kid who was given a treadmill for Christmas because the family was worried about their weight.

We may have positive memories of active play, sport, dance, and other movement activities in our early childhood, but by the time we reach middle school, most if not all of us become more aware of how bodies "stack up," where we fall along the body hierarchy, and whether or not we are part of an elite group. Here's a bit of Aaron's body story:

> As I became a teenager, I was spending time with my shirt off
> at summer camp and I noticed I didn't have a body like some
> of my friends. That my body just didn't look the same. And

then I really noticed it with athletics. I played volleyball in high school and I was an average player, maybe a little above average. Where I grew up, volleyball is the sport. All the athletes played volleyball. I remember in ninth grade trying to do everything I could to be a starter. To jump higher and do everything better. And there were improvements, but I realized there was no way I was going to athletically beat out my best friend, who was the starter. He was just better. Our bodies were different. He was smaller than I was, more defined, and no matter how much I did, I knew that my body was never going to be like his. And so that was what started this idea that my body is not elite. My body's not a starter body. My body is going to be on the bench. And there was nothing I could really do to change that. It sucked, it was a horrible feeling.

Here in the United States, one thing that makes it abundantly clear as to where we fall along the body hierarchy is the Presidential Fitness Test. With tremendous wit and humor, Aubrey Gordon and Michael Hobbes unpacked the history of the Presidential Fitness Test on their podcast, The Maintenance Phase.[6] Some of you won't be surprised to find out that it's a racket. What began in the 1950s as concern about children's fitness as it related to military prowess eventually became the White House Council on Health and Fitness (now known as the President's Council on Sports, Fitness and Nutrition) and the rollout of the first U.S. government fitness test, which was adopted by some states. In the late 1980s and early '90s, concern about TV time and the rise of the "obesity epidemic" prompted states to pass laws requiring that all kids have an annual fitness test. They eventually added body composition tests, including BMI and skinfold measurements, which were often done in front of peers (ugh!). It was a recipe for disaster, and for some kids, the start of their eating disorder. Aubrey Gordon says, "The President's Fitness Test presents itself as public health work, but what it is doing is ramping up weight stigma." Not surprisingly, a significant percentage of elementary school teachers report students crying during testing and high school teachers report witnessing humiliating test experiences. At the end of the episode, Hobbes reads from one research article that pretty much says it all: "there is compelling evidence that fitness test experiences do little to promote positive feelings about lifelong physical activity and fitness."

The Presidential Fitness Test led to the quantification of fitness, with its focus on competition, and awards going to those who scored in the 85th percentile or above. Basically, the kids who were already athletically inclined, while many kids walk away with trauma attached to movement and negative attitudes about this warped construct of fitness that persist well into adulthood.

The changes that come with puberty and sexuality increase thoughts about appearance, desirability, and attractiveness. There's the natural weight gain that gets problematized and pathologized. The amplified gender dysphoria for some trans and nonbinary kids. What was once a form of active play becomes a way of modifying the body, shrinking those curves, attaining six-pack abs or the coveted thigh gap. We move away from a subjective experience of the body and begin to view the body as something that must be tightly controlled. We buy into the "calories in/calories out" equation we are sold, and exercise is now a way to compensate for our food intake. Niva Piran says, "Post-puberty, joyful immersion and agency in physical activities are commonly replaced by compulsive, often joyless physical activities aimed at body alterations—such as weight loss or body sculpting—anchored in experiences of deficiency rather than agency."[7] Let's take a look at Melissa's story:

> *Like most humans, I get pleasure out of movement, but that got*
> *interrupted by diet culture at a relatively young age. I enjoyed*
> *playing sports and running and baseball just for the fun of it.*
> *But as I started to go into adolescence, there was a clear con-*

nection between movement, food, and body size. Movement and exercise became a tool to get to thinness. It became an obligation to do a certain way, a certain number of times a week, in order to achieve a certain size.

My relationship with fitness or just movement in general has been complicated over my entire life. Once I started to walk away from that whole idea of cosmetic fitness—which is a term I had not heard that I love now because that's totally what it is—and got closer to Health at Every Size, I almost didn't know what to do with myself around working out. I would still feel guilty for not working out. If I skipped today, then I'd try to make up for it the next time. I still had thoughts of working out to achieve a certain physical appearance. And I was missing physical movement. But if your only or primary experience with movement is in the context of diet culture or weight loss or health, it can be really disorienting going into fitness spaces and trying to do it from a different perspective.

I historically have loved going into gyms and lifting weights. But there was a time where I needed space to figure out what felt good to me. Do I like yoga? Do I really like lifting? I took a break from regular workouts because I felt like I was just on autopilot. So I stayed away for weeks at a time, which I thought I would never do. But I couldn't even bring myself to do it. I just didn't feel it. Everything had been so prescribed, I wasn't sure what I wanted.

For a time, I was just dancing at home. I love music. I love playing music at home. I was like, "This feels good to me. I'm going to dance until I'm done with it, and then I'm going to move on." Part of me reclaiming movement is that my exercise is less structured. I don't have specific weekly goals. Sometimes I go to the gym and lift weights, and sometimes I work out at home. I don't know what I'm going to do until I get there and I see how I feel. I just kind of let myself figure it out. I don't force myself into anything. I don't do the whole push thing anymore. I stop when I feel like I've had enough. I don't necessarily use a clock. I start when I start and I stop when I stop. It feels less restrictive now.

I enjoy movement. I like the way it feels to move my body. And movement is rarely connected to enjoyment and pleasure. You grow accustomed to not experiencing that while you're working out. Sometimes you check out just to get it done, like checking a box. Which I guess is fine sometimes. But I want people to realize that there's this huge possibility of pleasure and enjoyment in movement. It can look however it looks for you as an individual. And it's okay to take the space you need to figure it out.

I'm reclaiming fitness as something that connects me to myself. I choose movement that respects and accommodates my aches and pains instead of overriding them. I choose movement that is nourishing and not punishing. I choose movement that makes me feel the aliveness in my body. When I expand the definition of exercise, I can't fail. Whatever I choose will always be enough. I will always be enough.

Melissa's story is one example of what a relationship with movement might look like as we divest from diet culture (and toxic fitness culture) and explore various activities through Niva Piran's five dimensions of embodiment: body connection and comfort, desire, agency, attuned self-care, and subjective immersion.[8] She allowed for a lot of flexibility, with permission to adjust based on what felt good in the moment.

Exploring how dominant culture's ideas of health, ability, size, gender, age, and beauty have impacted your relationship with movement is an important part of your body story. The allure of the cosmetic fitness industry is that we can remake our body into something different and more desirable if we just work hard enough.

We wonder what your relationship with movement is like today. We know a grandiose plan for compensatory exercise is often part of The Cycle. A bad (body) day leads to thoughts like "Tomorrow I'll start working out at the gym two hours a day." We may be all in for a few days or weeks, feeling hopeful while we are in the honeymoon phase, and then the unsustainability of The Plan makes itself known. So the question is, how do you begin to decouple urgency and expectations from your idea of movement?

As Melissa's story highlights, sometimes The Plan is to resist the urge to make a plan and give ourselves time to sit in inaction until something that is genuinely ours shows up. In order to do that, we can't sit in inaction that's laden in shame. This compassionate form of inaction is about holding space, letting go, grieving, and seeing what needs to move through us in order for something new to be born.

There have been real barriers to making movement yours. In this time of compassionate inaction, you are making space for your personal movement philosophy to emerge from the depths of your own being, rooted in your own motivations and connected to what works best for you, your body, your personality, and your unique life.

While most if not all bodies benefit from and appreciate some movement every day, what that looks like will vary from person to person. There isn't a one-size-fits-all approach. There's nothing wrong with you or your body if you're not athletically inclined or don't strive to be. Some people aren't wired that way; and some of us don't need to believe there is an athlete (or a thin person!) inside just waiting to be discovered. That doesn't mean we can't find enjoyable ways to move our body that enhance our health and well-being. We may be happy with a leisurely trip to the park or prefer activities outside, like gardening. Others love running or an intense workout in the gym. Some will want to take classes or go on hikes with a group of people. Others prefer solitude. There's no right way to do this—and there's no mandate to do it, either. What you feel drawn to do, enjoy doing, and what you are able to do will change over the course of your lifetime. And it should change if you are listening to and honoring your body as it ages.

You see, the relationship with movement is constantly changing. There are times when we are in a routine and times when we are kicked out of our routine. Times when we have access and times when we don't. We experience health conditions that encourage us to move toward or away from certain activities. It's not a static experience. It will evolve and change with the complexity of real life, and the flexibility that our lives demand. It's your body and you get to figure out what you want your relationship with movement to be. It doesn't have to look like anybody else's.

So instead of an organized plan that just leads to another trip around The Cycle, what if the purpose of movement was to bring you into relationship with the living tissue, breathing lungs, beating heart of your body? What if it was centered around pleasure and provided opportunities to connect with your body and start trusting your own rhythms? What might movement rooted in self-nurturance or self-tending with gentle expectations look like? Here's what Angeline P. said when asked how their relationship with movement has evolved and changed doing Body Trust work:

> I move in ways that feel loving and not punishing toward my body. I tried scuba diving (being a fat person in a wet suit was a struggle of mine) and loved it. I have a kayak, stretch sometimes, dance, ride my bike and hike because all of these activities satisfy me and bring me joy. For a long time, I thought exercise was about changing my body. Now it's about enjoying all the amazing things I can do.

I.B. really loved going for long bike rides, especially in the mountains. He loved picking a challenging route and the sense of accomplishment that came at the end of the ride. On one particularly long ride, his body was really feeling pushed beyond his capacity, but he didn't stop. So when his body finally gave out, his feet were stuck in the toe clips and he fell over attached to his bike. After exploring the concept of doing activities *for and with* the body as opposed to *to and on* the body, he was able to start paying attention for the moments when his attitude toward the challenging work of riding his bike shifted away from what felt like a healthy push, and he could make the compassionate choice to get off the bike and either take a break or walk the rest of the way.

Just because an activity challenges you doesn't mean it's disordered or harmful. But when people do not like their bodies or they are disconnected from their bodies for any reason, there can be a risk of pushing past pain, ignoring body signals, or doing things with an element of self-harm. Your body isn't something that needs to be conquered. Physical therapist assistant and ACE-certified medical exercise specialist Ilya Parker says,

> *A lot of folks have this expectation that I, as the trainer, am to "punish" them for an hour. If they're not breathing heavier, feeling so much muscle tension, or their heart rate's not up—they think that they didn't really get a workout. When I first started my transition and moved into the exercise realm, I thought I was supposed to beat my body up. That's why I have a lot of chronic injuries now. That's what I saw other transmasculine people doing in all these YouTube videos by cis-aligned, aesthetically pleasing white trans men. I was legit that person puking in the bucket of sawdust and jumping right back into exercise—working out in the grungy garage gyms and just killing myself, until I knew better.*

For those of you who feel drawn to more strenuous forms of movement, the question is, how do you find your edge, where you feel challenged—it can even feel hard—but you aren't pushing so far that you are putting yourself at risk of injury? If you struggle with permission to take days to rest, or to listen to your body when it is injured, you may have a compulsive exercise disorder.

Meret Boxler, host of the podcast "Life. Unrestricted.," said, "When I was at my worst in my exercise addiction, I got compliments all around for my incredible fitness and my discipline, which only reinforced the problem. It took me a long time to speak up and tell them, 'I do this out of fear; I'm terrified of not doing it.'"

The National Eating Disorders Association defines compulsive exercise as "exercise that significantly interferes with important activities, occurs at inappropriate times or in inappropriate settings, or when the individual continues to exercise despite injury or other medical complications."[9] It often functions as a compensatory behavior to support efforts to regulate caloric intake and body size, or as permission to eat. It can also be used to numb emotions. And due to our pro-exercise and exertion culture, exercise compulsion is often rewarded and rarely recognized as harmful. The TV show *The Biggest Loser* is an endorsement for compulsive exercise. People are encouraged to exercise at extreme levels, often to the point of vomiting or passing out, all in the name of weight loss under the guise of "health promotion."

We wrote this chapter to help you divest from toxic ideas about fitness and reclaim a sense of agency so you can determine what feels best for you and your unique body moving forward. The exploration of movement through the lens of Body Trust presents an opening for befriending the body, getting below the neck, and coming home. When you adopt a Body Trust approach to movement, you:

* root movement in loving-kindness, gentle expectations, and weight neutrality

* do things *for and with* your body as opposed to *to and on* your body

* keep the focus on how various activities support your body and/or enhance your health and well-being

* move your body in ways that connect you to sensation, pleasure, and joy

* notice how it feels to move your body

* adjust activities based on your energy level and what sounds good to you/your body

* eat enough to fuel your activities

* avoid using activities for compensatory reasons

* can take days off to rest without feeling guilt or shame

* don't let fitness trackers override your rhythms and your own knowing

It can be hard to find a way back into movement that hasn't been touched by the fitness industry. Most gym environments collude with diet culture, uphold a fit aesthetic under the guise of health, and contribute to body shame. You may need to pause your gym membership and other activities you've been engaged in for a while to help you unhook. Your first step may be to increase your awareness of the ways a toxic fitness mindset shows up in your life and lay down the ideas and activities that are no longer serving you. Perhaps there are some items that you want to place on your grief altar to honor and acknowledge this transition.

Start with an intention to create opportunities for movement and see what unfolds. And give yourself permission to explore with grace. Movement can be confrontational, particularly if it has been a while since you've done an activity. It takes time to become conditioned to doing something—to build up strength, flexibility, and endurance. Don't be an asshole to yourself. Start slowly. This is your body and we trust your process.

BODY STORY
SUBMERGED

by Gabe Montesanti

I learned how to swim at the army base in Anchorage, where my mom worked when I was young. The pool was otherwise vacant, so the lifeguard had no choice but to watch as we splashed and played in the shallow water. This is one of my earliest memories. His stare didn't bother me—I had not yet learned to be self-conscious about the soft rolls of my legs or the way my tummy emerged from the water like a tortoiseshell when I floated on my back.

There are pictures from my baptism in the family photo albums. A man in green robes holds me up as I drip with holy water. In catechism class, I will learn that gluttony is a sin. In the years to come, I will gorge and force myself to throw up. I'll learn, over time, how to do this quietly, minimizing the splash, like a prestigious diver entering the water after three and a half rotations off the high dive.

I started swimming competitively at age nine. My body was strong, but by then I was preoccupied with the way my thighs looked as I sat on the metal benches before my races. Dad told me to scooch to the end of the bench so that the fat wouldn't get pushed up. He too was preoccupied with helping me be the smallest version of myself.

My mother's philosophy of food was informed by the fact she was a Weight Watchers leader. "Sometimes when you think you're hungry, you're really just thirsty for water," she would often say. It was a trick she had learned in class: fill your stomach with water to drown your hunger cues. Sometimes it worked. Sometimes it made me feel sick.

When I broke my first competitive swimming record at age ten, I tasted victory I wanted to gorge on. It didn't take long before I became obsessed with the times I needed to beat, doodling them in the margins of my science test and in the pages of my planner. I wrote them on the back of my hand in Sharpie the night before every swim meet and woke up with black marker stains all over my cheeks and legs.

It wasn't just that the water was a way to prove my worth: the swimming pool was also the only place my body didn't hurt. The pain was in both feet: a structural abnormality, the doctors said, that made it unbearable to support my own weight. I tried creams and orthopedics and pills. For a period of time, I attended the fifth grade with a cane. Eventually, a surgeon reconfigured the shape of both my feet using a plate and several screws.

Just as I denied my hunger for food, I also learned to deny my feelings for other women. That is, until I fell in love with the captain of my collegiate swim team at age eighteen. She enamored me, fascinated me. I still remember the way the chlorine lingered on her skin, tangled up in her bedsheets. When my mother found out we were dating, she said she could no longer eat, no longer breathe.

At my first Pride parade, I climbed into a fountain with all my clothes on. It was hot; I wanted to cool off, but it was also a sort of baptism. In a different time, I would've refused to go into the water, knowing that my drenched T-shirt would cling to my belly—that I wouldn't be able to hide.

When I was twenty-two, I joined the local roller derby team. I was attracted to the queerness, the physicality, the campiness. I thought I had traded swimming for derby, thought that I was done with the water—until I broke my leg. Suddenly I needed the water again as badly as I had when I was eleven, walking with a cane. My physical therapists instructed me to start walking again in neck-high water so that the weight of my body put less pressure on my healing bones.

In my first session with an anti-diet dietitian, she asked me what a basketball does in water. I thought it was a trick question. "It floats . . ." I said. She nodded emphatically. Then she mimed pushing the ball underwater. She told me that all these years of fighting with my body—trying to control my eating and my exercise was like holding the ball under with both hands.

"Takes a lot of work," she explained. "You can't move your hands even for a second or the ball will fly back up. But what would it look like to just let the ball float?"

The question came with such a sense of relief. I couldn't help but imagine how much more time and energy I would have if I wasn't focusing so hard on holding the ball under. I felt certain I would be drawing more, writing more, connecting with the wonderful people in my life.

It's not always easy to let the ball float. There are days I weigh myself or purge or work out until my vision goes black. But there are also days where I gently take my hands off the ball and let it rise to the surface of the water. I nourish myself. I eat when I am hungry. I move only for the joy of it. Those are my happiest days.

A year ago, I married my college swim team captain. When it's warm enough, we go to the community pool together, but we never race anymore. We sit poolside with our legs dangling in the cool water, laughing. I love watching the way the light warps and breaks in the water, dancing along the pool floor.

CHAPTER 11

Deepening Your Roots into Body Trust

For most humans, transformation does not seem achievable from the distant shores of another person's life. From far away, transformation looks like a miracle, or the result of magical powers possessed by the transformed person. Transformation is not magic. It's hard work. But it is also doable work. When we can see another person's labor toward their transformation, we know it is not some secret sauce but instead a daily commitment to a new way of life.[1]

—SONYA RENEE TAYLOR, from *The Body Is Not an Apology*

Here we are. You made it close to the end of this book. Whew. Or perhaps you've started and stopped a few times thinking, *No . . . it can't be true*. Only to find yourself days/weeks/months later thinking, *Well . . . maybe. Okay, maybe*. And then eventually going, *All right, now what did I do with that Body Trust book?* This is what the path to Body Trust looks like for many folks. This is The Reclamation. Danna Faulds reminds us:

> To take one step is courageous;
> to stay on the path day after day,
> choosing the unknown, and facing
> yet another fear, that is nothing
> short of grace.[2]

If you've made it this far in our book, that is nothing short of grace. Remember, reclaiming body trust is an ongoing, evolving process that is multifaceted and nonlinear, in part because you are doing this work in a toxic atmosphere. Just like fish are unaware they are in water, most people don't even stop to think and question what we've been socialized to believe about food, weight, bodies, and health. They don't even consider that there might, indeed, be another way.

We didn't write this book to be right. We wrote it because the dominant weight paradigm is harming people and this is what we've found to be truly healing in our twenty-plus years of clinical practice as a therapist and dietitian and sixteen-plus years working together, doing our own learning and unlearning as we create the language and philosophy that is Body Trust. Those of us who choose a different path are often "rejected, unrecognized, misunderstood, judged," as mystic L'Erin Alta writes in a poem about liberation called "It's Worth It." Some people may think you've joined a cult. Others will think you are in deep denial or that you lack discipline and self-control so you've decided to throw in the towel. Or it's "an excuse" to stay fat (insert eyeroll). We hope this book helps you build a solid foundation beneath you so it isn't as easy to get knocked off center and pulled away from the truth of your lived experience. The deeper your roots are in this work, the stronger the foundation and the more resilient you will be to handle various weather patterns in the atmosphere.

Body Trust is countercultural. While this movement began over fifty years ago, those of us choosing this path today would still be considered early adopters. Many don't even know a path like this exists. So when you share what you are learning here with people you know and love and trust, you will likely hear things like "that won't work" or "what about so-and-so, they've kept the weight off." This is because you are speaking a language that is foreign to them and new to you, and you may not have the words or the analysis to hold your ground and fully articulate what you are learning.

When you are fairly new in your own process and understanding of Body Trust, comments from family, friends, coworkers, and medical providers can make you second-guess yourself, so you might protect it for a while. You know your truth. You've learned from your lived experience. And now that you've reached this part of the book, you may know that you can't go back even though you don't know how to go forward, which is where this work often begins. When people arrive on our doorstep, they know, on some level, that what they are doing isn't working. They are tired. There is some acknowledgment that they can't keep doing what they've always done and yet they do not know another way. And the fear of body changes and weight gain can stop people in their tracks.

We cannot tell you what will happen with your weight when you divest from diet culture and come home to yourself. We don't know how long you've been dieting or how restrictive your food intake has been in recent weeks/months/years. We don't know how much healing work you've had access to. All we know is that one of three things will happen when you do this work: you will gain weight, you will lose weight, or your weight will stay the same. This is probably not what you want to hear, and if we didn't tell the truth, we'd be no different than most programs or professionals you've sought out for help with this. Nobody really knows where your body wants to be, where it is comfortable. The white dude that created the BMI certainly didn't know. The lady at

Jenny Craig didn't know. Your doctor doesn't know, nor does the personal trainer. WW and Noom don't know. But your body knows. And we trust your body to sort out the weight.

In this work, you are rebuilding trust that was whittled away by the cycle of disordered eating and the subsequent body distrust. The process of rebuilding trust with food, body, and self is not all that different from how we rebuild trust in any relationship in our life when it is broken, so take a moment to explore this question before you continue reading:

> *If you lost trust in another relationship in your life, what would you need in place to rebuild it?*

Years ago, we asked our Body Trust Community about this, and here are some of our favorite responses:

* Time and love, *lots* of love

* If there is no love, you wouldn't even want to try

* Transparency, a willingness to be vulnerable, and clear (and realistic) expectations paired with ongoing communication

* Forgiveness

* An acknowledgment that trust was broken in the first place

* Space for anger and hurt to show up

* A lot of listening

* A willingness to surrender to what the journey brings along the way

* Positive experiences in the new direction to help me know it's real

* Connecting to something bigger than what was broken, and focusing energy and efforts on that

* Remembering that there is a deeper learning happening inside

* Faith in the process; believing in ourselves

* Actual change of behavior—not just words, promises, intentions, or gestures

* Releasing fear and choosing love, over and over again

* Grace to experience pain along the journey of rebuilding and repairing

Body Trust is repair work. And just like when you've lost trust in any relationship in your life, trust can be broken in a matter of seconds, and it takes much longer to get it back. You don't just say, "Okay, I'll trust you now." John Gottman's research on approaches to relationships shows that attunement and small consistent acts over time reintroduce trust, not conditional acts or large-scale gestures.[3] When it comes to Body Trust, this trust is reciprocal—you are working on attuning to, discerning, and trusting the ways your body talks to you as well as trusting your body's ability to regulate your weight, and your body is working on trusting that enough food will be eaten consistently and predictably. This requires open communication between you and your body: checking in regularly, acknowledging what is needed, and responding as best you can, given your capacity and resources. Sometimes you listen to your body's signals and follow the wisdom; sometimes you are unable to. Either way, you have an experience of tuning in and noticing what happens next. The information gathered over time, with curiosity and kindness, will help you rebuild trust with yourself and your body, and you'll have a stronger belief in your ability to handle whatever comes your way.

Writer and coach Sam Dylan Finch shared this in an Instagram post:

"Why should I trust my body?" isn't the question, really. It's this: Who told you that you couldn't? When did you begin to doubt your own resilience and adaptability? When did your body become a target instead of an ally? When did punishing your body become your default orientation to your own gorgeous being? . . . All my body wanted was for me to live. My eating disorder wanted me not to exist. I'm going to trust the parts of me that fiercely cling to life—and I'll remain grateful, receptive, and willing as I relinquish the illusion of control so that I can live a vibrant life. Unrestricted, unapologetic. Full.[4]

We use the metaphor (and image) of a young tree working on establishing its roots to describe the phases we move through as we rebuild trust with ourselves and our bodies. Working with the various concepts, ideas, tools, and practices in the tree is what will deepen your roots into body trust. We chose this image to illustrate how the various phases have influence over the others and "get the wheels turning." Many of the concepts in the tree have been explored in one way or another earlier in the book, but let's revisit them again here because they may help you to see how this all fits together.

Engage in Heady Exploration of Alternative Paradigms

The first step, as we mentioned earlier, is acknowledging that you cannot go back to what you've always done even though you don't necessarily know how to move forward. As we reckon with the fact that what we've been doing isn't working for us, the next thing people usually do is immerse themselves in books, podcasts, and programs to learn more about alternatives to diet culture and connect the dots between weight science, eugenics, anti-fatness, and anti-Blackness. (We've got lots of recommendations on our website.) Folks need time to intellectualize it, but intellectualizing it is not the same as embodying it. Over the years, we've noticed how many of the participants in our workshops and retreats have read a lot of books in this arena and listened to all the podcasts (some could write a damn book about it!), but they struggle to take actions that will help them fully embody a Body Trust philosophy in their life. They may believe in and want this for everyone else, and still be restricting and restraining food themselves, secretly thinking there's a different set of rules for "people like me." This work isn't done until all people and all bodies are included, and that means you too!

Body Trust is something that takes practice. A heady exploration will get you only so far. Imagine that you wanted to learn to play a musical instrument. You could read every book ever written about that instrument. You could watch a thousand how-to videos of people playing the instrument. You might play a killer air guitar! But if you never picked up the instrument and practiced playing it, you wouldn't expect to be able to play it. And when you first play, it is awkward, bumpy, clunky. It sounds janky. But if you keep showing up to practice playing the instrument, you won't have to think about every single little thing you are doing. With time and practice, it would start to sound better and playing would feel more natural to you.

If there is one thing we know for certain will help you sink your roots more deeply into Body Trust, it is risk-taking and working the edges of your comfort zone. You'll need to get curious about what happens when you say yes; what happens when you say no, or not now. It won't always be pretty. You will fall down, kick/scream/cry on the ground before you get back up, dust yourself off, and try again. This is what it looks like to practice. Don't look too far ahead because you'll get overwhelmed. Don't spend too much time thinking about the past because you'll feel defeated. Take it one step, one eating episode, one day at a time. Let each moment be a blank slate. With practice, there will come a time in your Body Trust practice where not doing it will be harder than doing it.

Explore Your Body Story

As you read in chapter 2, exploring your body story is a powerful catalyst for reclaiming body trust. When you investigate and shine a light on the experiences you've had living in your body, something deep within begins to shift. The part of you that's been minimized and silenced by dominant culture begins to show up, speak up, take up space, and reclaim what is rightfully yours. Your body story is more powerful than you may know.

Delving into your body story through the lens of Body Trust gives you an opportunity to take control of the narrative and rewrite the ending instead of having the story narrated for you by the mouthpieces with power who believe they know better. The narrative changes from "What the hell is wrong with me?" to "My body is not the problem and this struggle is not my fault." We turn the tables and authentically ask, "What the hell is wrong with the world?" Writer Rebecca Solnit says, "The ability to tell your own story, in words or images, is already a victory, already a revolt."

Illuminate the Pattern of Coping You Developed to Survive

It is hard to disrupt patterns when you are not aware of them, when you cannot see their cyclical nature. So another phase of deepening your roots into body trust is to begin to familiarize yourself with the pattern of coping you've developed to survive. Begin by naming it when you see it. Most people first become aware of The Cycle when they are Making a Plan. You can walk it back from there. What was happening before you were planning? How were you feeling? What were you doing?

Take time to get to know what thoughts, feelings, sensations, and behaviors arise in your pattern, and how other people in your life intersect with it. Look for where shame shows up within the cycle, and also where restriction lives in your thoughts as well as your behaviors. Shame and restriction are always a part of The Cycle, no matter what you are calling The Problem (your body, your food choices, overeating, emotional eating, attuned eating, etc.). What do your plans for solving the problem sound like? How long do your plans usually last? What happens next?

The weapons of shame, tough love, discipline, and conditional self-regard add fuel to the fire and speed up The Cycle. This work is not about becoming better behaved; it is about growing in trust and understanding of your inner workings, your well-honed and wise patterns, and the way internalized oppression and dominance have worked through you. Kindness offers a path forward and an entry point to a relationship with yourself that you want to be in and can therefore sustain. We've got lots of good resources on our website to help you explore your cycle and you might revisit chapter 3.

Grieve, and Then Grieve Some More

There's so much to grieve in this work that we name it twice in our Body Trust framework. As you do a heady exploration, explore your body story, and illuminate the pattern of coping you've developed to survive, you're likely going to get pissed off. And instead of blaming yourself, the anger you've long internalized will start to be externally directed toward the things that should rightfully be blamed—anti-fat bias, transphobia, sexism and misogyny, racism, classism, healthism, ableism.

Make space for the grief by creating a grief altar. As you move through the various stages of grief, you will more clearly see what's been put upon your body that was never yours to begin with. You'll develop some reverence for your body—the keeper of your story, the one that has shown up for you, day after day, despite all it has been through with you. Body Trust participant LMT writes:

> *My Body is My Body, for better or worse. It has been with me*
> *every step of my seventy-plus years life on Earth. If it could*

have, My Body would have divorced itself from me many years ago. Instead, it has been loyal to me and stuck with me through times of disgust, shame, abuse, hatred, deprivation, malnutrition, and lack of any sense of security of knowing what it could expect from me from one moment to the next. Hindsight, while I now grieve all of these various abuses and years lost to Body Obsession, Diet Culture, Fatphobia, Capitalism, and all of the other by-products of our Patriarchal Society, I now also recognize that I would not be alive today writing My Body's Story had I not manipulated it as a means of coping throughout the various stages of my life. Yes, it is time that I give voice to My Body for all of its unwavering loyalty that has brought me to this point in my life.

Divest from Diet Culture

Before the concepts in this book can firmly take root, you will need to get down in the trenches and dig out the old roots, the invasive species, all the ways you have been conditioned from an early age to think about bodies, gender, beauty, food, fitness, health, and weight. According to Wikipedia, culture is "an umbrella term which encompasses the social behavior and norms found in human societies, as well as the knowledge, beliefs, arts, laws, customs, capabilities, and habits of individuals in these groups."

Weight is a normative discontent. Restricting and restraining food for the purpose of controlling our bodies is a normative behavior. Exercising to perfect our bodies under the guise of health is a normative behavior. Once you wake up to the hustle that diet (and dominant) culture promotes, you will start to recognize it in people and places that were undetectable before: the juice cleanse at the yoga studio, your doctor telling you not to diet but to focus on a "healthy lifestyle," and the celebrities and people with huge platforms sharing their diet and exercise plans and talking about what works for them (um, mostly privilege and genetics). We wrote an entire chapter on divestment—chapter 4, "Divesting from Diet Culture"—that will be useful to revisit.

Body Trust is an invitation to let go of what no longer serves you. Here's what L.W. had to say about this phase of the work:

> *It's been a bit like unschooling for me—I'm allowing myself a "detox" period where I have no rules whatsoever. I eat what I want. I move how I want. And I pay attention to how I feel and make note of it. I've lived by the rules of diet culture, and then wellness culture for nearly all of my life, and before I can get to body trust, I have to let all of that energy unwind out of me—and a part of how I'm doing that is by wholeheartedly embracing an energy of no-rules.*

Divesting from diet culture will allow you to begin rooting into something more deeply nourishing of your entire being.

Allow for Pleasure and Satisfaction

Reclaiming pleasure is an act of resistance in a culture that has made indulgence a "dirty word." Pleasure takes up space and says, "I'm here." It is not a shrinking back, but rather an expansion and expression of ourselves. We believe pleasure, in the absence of shame and guilt, heals.

Satisfaction is a crucial ingredient in your efforts to heal your relationship with food and body. In more recent editions of *Intuitive Eating*, Evelyn Tribole and Elyse Resch write: "it has become more evident that finding satisfaction in eating is the driving force of this process."[5] Satisfaction is the state of being fulfilled or content. We wonder if the hustle has ever led to experiences of fulfillment or contentment. Has it ever been good enough? Is there ever a place you've arrived and thought, "I'm good now"? If so, how long did/does that feeling last? When does the line or target get slippery? Does it keep moving? Do you ever get to rest? When does hypervigilance end? And if it does end, what happens next?

Allowing for pleasure and satisfaction is not about being in a heady state of ecstasy at all times, but rather learning how to sense when something is good for you and to be able to feel what "enough" is. When you increase your connection to the erotic—a deeper way of knowing—you will discover what you really like, what turns you on, what lights you up, what deeply nourishes you, as well as what turns you off, and what doesn't do it for you. Start to pay attention to whether or not you like what you are eating. Do you like how you are spending your free time? The activities you are doing? The people you hang out with? Who and what in your life nourishes your sense of worthiness? Even if you can't always get what you want, you deserve to know what you feel drawn to as well as what makes you feel good.

Reconnect with Your Needs and Boundaries

Dominant culture chips away at our embodied knowledge and overrides our boundaries. The ways we learn to cope with food—and leave our bodies—have been about learning to survive because our boundaries, our bodies, and our own knowing are not being respected. When we are divesting from diet culture, we need boundaries to protect our healing process as we find new ways to inhabit our own being. You may have never told anyone about your experiences with disordered eating, and this is the first time you are naming and sharing this part of your story. As a result, you may be vulnerably asking for less stigmatizing conversation about your body or all bodies. Or asking people to reduce diet and healthist conversations in your presence, even if they don't fully "get it." People in your life, including your medical providers, may not be able to meet you respectfully in your process. Your boundaries may look like not talking about it (yet) or asking for conversations to stop or not happen altogether. It can be refusing to step on the scale and asking your doctor not to talk to you about food or your weight without your permission.

A boundary is a limit or a line between you and someone or something else. It may be a no or a not yet or a not now. Boundaries help us define our capacities, limits, and consent and are the expression of our ever changing yeses and noes. Whether we know it or not, we set boundaries all the time:

> No, I don't want another cup of coffee.
>
> Yes, I am ready to start.
>
> No, I don't need the extended warranty.
>
> That's enough, thanks.

Some of our boundaries come from within—they are instinctive or intuitive—and some come in response to how we are understood or interpreted by the culture. They exist whether you are aware of them, have permission to speak them, or choose to assert them. They simply are what they are, though they aren't always easy to name or express. Here are a few gentle reminders:

* You get to be separate from other people. Boundaries can help you connect with your edges: where you end and others begin.

* Boundary setting is both self-advocacy and staying in alignment with yourself.

* Trust that setting boundaries can be a bid for more closeness and connection.

Ultimately, our boundaries improve our relationship with ourselves and with others. Prentis Hemphill, founder of The Embodiment Institute, says, "Boundaries are the distance at which I can love you and me simultaneously." We are better at love and compassion when we know where we want our boundaries to be. We are in general more curious about other people's boundaries, too. We become better at consent.

You might find it harder to take risks in your healing process when your boundaries feel more porous. Personal agency is a part of how you move more deeply toward honoring the needs that arise from owning your lived experience. In her book *Pleasure Activism*, adrienne maree brown writes, "Your strong and solid no makes way for your deep, authentic yes . . . by practicing saying no, you will cultivate a yes that is rooted in having agency, having power, and having respect for your boundaries."

Boundaries are also a central part of our justice work. In the book *Living in Liberation: Boundary Setting, Self-Care and Social Change*, Cristien Storm writes: "Boundary work is just as much about negotiating and asking for what we want and need as what we don't want and don't need. To this end, if we are working towards not just our own individual safety but towards changing the conditions in which people are not safe or are harmed, boundaries are about imagining radical possibilities as much as responding to events in the present."

Here's how to set a boundary:

* Name the behavior, pattern, concern. Taking time to try to specifically name the thing you want to change is a process. Examples: Mentioning your body size, touching you without asking, talking about a diet in front of you, weighing at the doctor's office, discussing your food choices, disregarding your no.

* Give a directive. These are best if they are free of judgment, blame, and shame. For example: "Next time, could you ask first?" versus "You never think to ask, what's wrong with you?" Cristien says there are positive directives and command directives. A positive directive might sound like, "Let's try again after we take a break." A command directive could be,

"You aren't listening to me. I am stopping this conversation." People are often not paying as much attention to us as we imagine or want them to be, so we often need to reinforce boundaries.

* Practice repeating the directive, like a broken record. Instead of getting pulled into justifying your reasoning, it can be helpful to lean on repeating your directive over and over again.

* End the interaction. It may be verbal or nonverbal, but make an ending—a punctuation mark—on the interaction to clearly state you are done and that is that.[6]

Your healing process and your Body Trust practice need your boundaries to continue. We wonder what you would like to protect in your Body Trust practice?

Redefine What Healing Looks and Feels Like

We encourage you to resist the urge to make Body Trust the next plan for how you are going to finally fix your body (it does happen!). The whole point of Body Trust is to trust your body to sort out the weight. This work is about healing, not fixing, so the old views of progress will not be useful here.

When you've read more books, explored your body story, and worked with some of the other concepts discussed in this chapter, you'll start to notice subtle shifts happening in your relationship to food, eating, movement, and your body. It can be a slow unraveling, and over time you'll see the fruits of your labor. Many weight loss programs sell quick fixes. Urgency is a characteristic of white supremacy culture, so keep asking yourself this question we learned from nationally recognized diversity, equity, and inclusion strategist Nicole Lee: "How do I do urgent work without urgency?" Remember trust is something that erodes fairly quickly but takes much longer to get back. Give yourself the space for something new to emerge.

We want you to identify other ways of knowing that our Body Trust approach is "working for you." The first thing you might notice is that you're using the word "notice" a lot, ha! More awareness of the thoughts that flood your mind when you are making decisions about what to eat or the way food and eating feels when you are dining with certain people. When you start to get enough to eat more consistently, you'll notice that you aren't thinking about food as much. You may enjoy food more, sit with less guilt or shame after eating, and be able to eat what you want in social situations without apology or excuses. The frequency and severity of your binges will lessen. You'll know what triggers bad (body) days and won't feel totally tanked by them. They may pull you under but for shorter periods of time, and you'll bounce back more quickly. You may have more pleasurable experiences moving your body, and less resistance to exploring different activities.

Shifting away from the outcome-oriented thinking of diet culture means our intentions and hopes become more personal and less oriented toward how we look—and what people think—to what makes us feel more at home in our bodies. Dominant cultural ideas tend to limit our imagination about how we talk about health and wellness, what is possible, and what we want to explore. If health and wellness are important to you, giving yourself some time and space to heal will help you find practices rooted in agency, sufficiency (enoughness), and what works in your unique life. It may be hard to imagine something fun, new, and exciting as you are just divesting. Your imagination will start doing its thing the more space you have. You can trust in that.

In the first part of the book, we explored The Rupture. How the seeds for a complicated relationship with food and body are planted early and begin to take root. How they get reinforced over the course of our childhood and adolescence, and puberty is the time when so many of us become firmly vested. The Hustle keeps us trapped in an endless cycle that has been about survival in a toxic world. Understanding the causes and conditions that create and maintain a traumatic and oppressive atmosphere is a vital part of the reclamation. Ruth King, founder of the Mindful of Race Institute, says, "There's a dance of dominance and subordination that perpetuates and fuels the clouds in the atmosphere, and all of us can relate to some degree of being traumatized by this dance of dominance and subordination at the collective level."

Exploring your body story uncovers all that has come between you and being at home in your body. Our hope is that this book has helped you understand your social conditioning, your indoctrination, how those early seeds were planted, how you lost trust with yourself and your body. And as you have a clearer vision of what has brought you to this point—sometimes a tipping point—you move into The Reckoning. There's so much to come to terms with and grieve. You are letting go of the navigation tools you've used to survive in a culture of domination. The culture isn't going to give you permission to trust your body. It's yours to reclaim. You may look away for a bit and try another plan. And then you remember how exhausting it is, that you just can't do it. As you illuminate the pattern of coping that's helped you survive, you begin to think maybe this struggle really isn't your fault. So you return to this work, this book. You may straddle for a while, with one foot in diet culture and the other in Body Trust. You wander and return; forget and remember, and all the while, the pattern or cycle you've been in is evolving and shifting. As you continue the work of divestment and pull your roots out of diet culture, The Cycle will have less of a hold on you. All the reading you've done in your heady exploration starts to click. You more consistently give yourself permission to eat. You let pleasure and satisfaction become a guidepost. You redefine what healing looks and feels like for *you*. And through the risks you take and the experiences you collect over time, you are reconnecting with your needs and boundaries, and become better equipped to celebrate your yeses and honor your noes.

The Foundations of Body Trust we introduced in the beginning of this book can help throughout all phases of this work. They are a set of key practices or roots to help you stick with this work throughout all these various phases so you can sink more deeply into it:

* Work the edges of your comfort zone

* Look and listen with kindness and curiosity

* Go for a C- (as opposed to an A)

* Locate yourself and widen the lens

* Find community and share your process

* Honor your self-preservation practices

We wonder how these six foundations have helped as you've read the book. Which concepts have you found yourself leaning into again and again? And what do you feel drawn to now?

Navigating a Bad (Body) Day

Something we haven't yet talked about in this book, and we know you'll likely need as you deepen your roots into Body Trust, is some help dealing with bad (body) days—days when you feel especially bad about your body or really feel the pull to make a plan to restrict food. While someone with a strong Body Trust practice is not immune from having bad (body) days, they have the analysis and tools to skillfully navigate these days without getting sucked back into harmful societal constructs and restrictive or compensatory behaviors. Here are some strategies for you to consider. Notice what speaks to *you*.

Acknowledge that this feeling is temporary. Most of the people we work with recognize that how they feel about their body can vary widely from day to day, or hour to hour. They can go to bed feeling neutral about their body and wake up the next morning feeling deep disgust. The body doesn't change significantly in short periods of time, but how we *feel* about our bodies does. So remember that the shame or discomfort you are experiencing ebbs and flows. Tomorrow is a new day and it might not even take that long for the feeling to change.

Get curious about what else might be going on. When we are distracted by the hustle, we lose access to language that describes our emotional world—our inner life—and we adopt the language of food and fat.[7] Our body becomes the scapegoat. Instead of recognizing our anger, we direct that anger toward our body. Instead of feeling anxious about the big deadline at work, we feel anxious about our size. Instead of feeling sad because we had a terrible fight with our partner, we think about a plan to control food and our body. Widen the lens and ask yourself: What would I be sitting with (feeling or thinking) right now if I weren't preoccupied with my food/body? What is going on in my life to make me want to focus on my body? Did I have a bad dream? Is my period due? Am I exhausted or overwhelmed? What else might be going on here?

Find a mantra to repeat to yourself. "This is temporary." "This is me. I am worthy because I breathe." "This is my body, this is where I live." "Every ounce is sacred." "I am more than my body." "My body is not a project or problem to be solved." Say it over and over in your head or out loud. Write it on Post-it Notes and stick it on every mirror in the house.

I will not let patriarchy, capitalist oppressive culture win.
I will not give my body and worth to a culture
that offers nothing in return.

—**Body Trust participant SHENA J.**

Avoid body checking behaviors. Standing in front of the mirror naked and scrutinizing yourself, weighing or taking measurements, feeling for bones/fatness, and comparing your body to others or in pictures past and present are just a few of the ways people body check. Take down or cover up your mirrors. Change your clothes if they are making you uncomfortable. Smash the scale or put it somewhere it is hard to access. Be aware of the pull toward these behaviors, and minimize opportunities to scrutinize, pathologize, or blame your body.

No fixin', no fixin', no fixin'! Bad body thoughts put you at a crossroad: you can choose to be compassionate and mindful, or you can make yet another unsustainable plan rooted in shame and deprivation. We suggest the former. Plans are always temporary fixes, even if your hope is that they will last forever. So resist the urge to make a plan. Notice thoughts like "Tomorrow I'll start going to the gym in the morning," "I'm only going to eat salads today," "I'll skip dinner," or "I've really got to stop eating sugar." Many in our community say it helps to remember what life was really like on their plans: how miserable they were, how crazy they felt around food, that they felt even worse without Body Trust. If right now, at this moment, you can't live without a plan, then plan for radical, weight-neutral self-care (that's self-care for the sake of self-care). Set realistic expectations for yourself. Perfectionism rears its head when we are feeling most vulnerable and worn out. Minimize expectations, maximize nurturing.

Name the systems of oppression that have infiltrated your consciousness and your body without your consent. Seeing our own body as the problem lets the culture, institutions, and structures that cause harm off the hook. So much of this work is externalizing and unlearning the dominance and oppression we've internalized. When we recognize and name how anti-fat bias, misogyny, patriarchy, ableism, white supremacy, transphobia, and other forms of oppression operate within us and cause us to blame our bodies and pathologize others' bodies, we can externalize those forces, and put the blame where it belongs. There is incredible power in asking questions like, Who profits from my belief that my body is a problem? Who is making money off my shame? Whose shit is this? And then say to yourself:

"I will not take what is not mine."

Honor, normalize, feel, and express your anger. Anger is an emotion that alerts us to harm and injustice. When we don't allow ourselves to be transformed by our anger, that emotion stays trapped in our bodies, gets internalized, and can increase anxiety and self-blame. We absolutely can experience, feel, and express anger and our hurt without resorting to aggression or harming others. Put on some heavy metal and dance it out, shake your fists at the wall, scream at the sky, punch a pillow, stomp your feet, give it to the earth, take a boxing class, write it out.

Have compassion for the ways you are still healing from the experiences in your body story. So many things make us feel betrayed by our bodies. Social constructs of gender, race, beauty, health, and weight. Chronic illness, infertility, and other health issues. Medical weight stigma, food insecurity, the ways our family of origin related to our body and their own bodies—all have a big impact on us. These wounds can flare up and need tending throughout our lifetime. Wanting things to be different than they are is one of the greatest sources of human suffering. Sometimes the question is: How do I soften when life invites me to harden? How do I not cling so tightly to something that I want so badly so I can see and experience it all with an open hand instead of a closed fist?

Your work, ultimately, on bad (body) days, is to extend to yourself the same grace and compassion you'd extend to everybody else. Perhaps lean on this loving-kindness phrase from Anna Guest-Jelley of Curvy Yoga:

> May I greet my body with gentleness.
>
> May I soften when life invites me to harden.
>
> May I listen to my intuition with wisdom and trust it with ease.
>
> May I appreciate my body a little more in this moment, just as it is.

We asked our beloved Body Trust Community, "What helped you sink your roots more deeply into Body Trust?" Here's what they shared with us:

* Following people who embrace these ideas. Seeing images of other people who celebrate, own, respect, rock, and care for their bodies is so healing.

* Patience and the C- work ethos.

* Learning from this community, letting go of what society expects from me, trying to think of other things besides my body and appearance.

* Going to a clothing-optional beach, wearing fun funky clothes, eating as I please and stopping when satisfied.

* Being honest with others about my experience and setting boundaries for myself.

* Seeing the systems behind my desire to lose weight. Looking at who makes the rules before we decide whether to follow them.

* Regular reminders from people I follow, such as the weekly Body Trust emails.

* Following other fat people on social media . . . seeing their pictures and their pride and seemingly lack of shame. Listening to anti-diet podcasts.

* Talking about my weight in a matter-of-fact way, not in a funny way or pretending that I'm not fat or that I don't know I'm fat, i.e., trying not to be ashamed.

* Having a journal to look back on or a friend or therapist to remind you of where you started.

* A desire to be truly free, to live my life whole and no longer broken. A deep knowing inside myself that everything was not okay.

* Giving myself space to pay attention to how I feel and what I need. Online community to help me change my thinking and give me models. Feeling into all that my body can do!

We hope reading this chapter along with what some of our Body Trust participants shared with us helps you to envision a path forward. Take what you feel ready to take; leave the rest for another person, or another time and place in your healing. Not everything we've written about in this chapter or this book will resonate, and it will be overwhelming to try to do it all at once. We encourage you to stay curious about where the resistance shows up. That may be the juiciest part of this work, where you'll find the most fruit for your labor. Maybe don't go for the hardest thing first. You certainly don't need to jump in with both feet. In fact, it's rare for people to show up to this work completely ready and all in. It's something most have to put in the pipe and smoke for a while.

We wonder what appeals to you right now based on your lived experience. What concepts and ideas do you feel drawn toward? Where might you begin? What's the next step?

We believe this work is for every body. Every. Single. One. And that includes you.

We encourage you to let the work be radical, from the roots, pulling up.

CHAPTER 12

Making Your Healing Bigger Than You

If you have come to help me you are wasting your time.
But if you have come because your liberation is bound up
with mine, then let us work together.

—ABORIGINAL RIGHTS ACTIVISTS FROM QUEENSLAND, AUSTRALIA

We hope, as you find yourself at the end of this book, you feel clearer as to why you have struggled to feel at home in your body. We hope you are shifting your focus to externalizing the shame, blame, and fatphobia that has contributed to the endless hustle of perfecting food and your body. We hope you are beginning to hold for yourself how this struggle has not been your fault. Bodies do not come with owner's manuals, but they do come with familial and cultural narratives (negative and some positive) that we learn prior to our ability to individuate. We imagine you are very clear on who has and still is profiting off this in your life. We also know this deep reckoning is often catalytic for people to understand that if it is happening to you, it has happened to more people than you. And that your healing process can extend beyond individual therapist or dietitian offices or a self-help book. As Nicola Haggett, a Body Trust Provider, writes: "Body Trust is both a personal journey *and* a political one—we can't unlearn body shame without exploring the cultural narratives that have contributed to and benefited from our shame." Moving beyond body shame is a political act that can influence more than "your one wild and precious life."[1]

A participant in one of our programs said it this way, "I try to imagine the world I want to live in (for example, a world of body acceptance), and I do what I can to live in that world as if it's already here. This happens in little moments and choices, like wearing or eating this or that, but those moments and choices feel big."

One way we dismantle structures is to divest personally from them. We have the power to collapse systems if we include ourselves in the process. This process is about healing and reclaiming body trust. It is also about changing the world, living from inclusion, and being audacious about belonging. One of the foundations of Body Trust is to locate yourself. Who are you in this? We know you believe in body trust for your mom, your kids, the neighbors, your friends, the Noom and WW coaches, the guy selling weight loss who won't deal with his history of disordered eating, your favorite influencers, and on and on. And who else? Who needs it more than you? How can your presence in this movement be about creating conditions for communion?

It takes time to get there, though. As we have said, people come and go from this type of healing work, remembering and forgetting. Trying and then going back to the comfort and safety of restriction and restraint. Trying and half-assing a new lifestyle plan. We know. We see you. It's okay if it takes time, but the truth of it is that we need your healing to not feel so optional when a paradigm shift is deeply needed in the world. And we can't forget that "No one asked your permission to put toxic thoughts about your body in your head," writes Emily Nagoski, PhD, in her book *Come As You Are*. "No one asked for your permission before they started planting the toxic crap. They didn't wait until you could give consent and then say, 'Would it be okay with you if we planted the seeds of body self-criticism and sexual shame?' Chances are, they just planted the same things that were planted in their gardens, and it never even occurred to them to plant something different."

And they did. They filled your head with bullshit. And you have had to make your way knowing the general public bought it all, too. What an incredible racket. What a bunch of lies to defy. Which is why your positionality—your identities and privileges—matter in this work. Understanding how your positionality has been a part of the body hierarchy is the work. It is why we are here. We must learn to reckon with the truth of this—that our participation or our turning away impacts the potential freedom for others. We can spend our whole lives in great pain about our body size and still experience the privilege of having a small, white, cisgender, able body in this culture. Choosing the safety and security of the plan is about surviving the present moment. Choosing something different is about the conditions we want to create, discover, or reclaim for ourselves, future generations, and the world at large. There's a lot we hold because this paradigm represents the complexity of all that we are, collectively. The third point in the Fat Liberation Manifesto—published by activists back in 1979—reads, "WE see our struggle as allied with the struggles of other oppressed groups against classism, racism, sexism, ageism, financial exploitation, imperialism and the like."[2] These differences in experience, even with the presence of great pain, are why the pain is possible in the first place. The reinforcement of a body hierarchy has to be our shared work to end.

When asked what keeps them going, a Body Trust participant shared the following:

> *Knowing that if I want this same sense of trust for everyone, it needs to start with me. I can only create acceptance of others to the extent that I do it for myself. I am deeply committed to collective liberation, so this work needs to start with my own divestment from systems that oppress bodies.*

This movement needs all of you, not just the part of you that wants freedom for everyone else. When we include ourselves in the process toward body liberation, we contribute to the movement. When we ground our healing in our story, we increase our agency and our voice. Once we've developed deeper roots in our Body Trust practice, it becomes easier to speak up and advocate for a body-compassionate and weight-inclusive world. And when we speak for a cause, our commitment to the cause strengthens. This work happens inside of us and out in the world. "When it comes to social change, belonging is at both an individual and a collective level," says Sebene Selassie, author of *You Belong*. This is a vision of a larger transformation.

bell hooks reminds us, "Rarely, if ever, are any of us healed in isolation. Healing is an act of communion."[3] What if your healing was never meant to be an individualized and private event? Maybe that is one reason things haven't been working? Collectively, we do need to get to the root of why eating disorders are notoriously long healing processes and treatment is not working well for most. What would be different or possible if you knew there was a fat-affirming community that wasn't marginalized as you worked to heal? What if you knew that the treatment community understood how anti-fatness is rooted in anti-Blackness? And that gender expansion was not for only a few brave and honest souls? And that the guides you relied on for your healing process had lived experiences similar to your own? And coping wasn't pathologized? And you were invited to externalize what should have never been internalized? What would healing be like for you? How would that differ from your experience now? How does this idea of healing as communion feel?

You may remember how one of the five dimensions of embodiment from Niva Piran's research was agency, both physical and voice.[4] When we have ruptures in our embodiment, we are less likely to believe in our ability to contribute, succeed, and make a difference. When we are disconnected from our bodies, our voices go underground. Part of the reclamation is regaining access to our voice; we speak up and advocate both for ourselves and for people who are pushed to the margins. Agency helps us show up and support the fat liberation movement. Using your voice for truth, difficult conversations, and advocacy will move you more deeply into this work because, again, when we speak for a cause, it strengthens our resolve.

Niva Piran, through her research on embodiment, identified "social power and relational connections" as one domain of social experiences that shapes the quality of embodied lives. The following protective factors that support embodiment are continually left out of eating disorder and body image research and curriculums:

* Freedom from stigma, prejudice, and harassment

* Access to resources

* Freedom from body-based harassment

* Freedom from appearance-based social power

* Empowering relationships that provide acceptance, validation, and role modeling

* Membership in equitable communities[5]

How do we begin to think of this work as a community effort, not a strictly individual one? Where we work toward relational constructs instead of self-contained individualism? And what does moving in that direction immediately do for your hurting and unhealed parts? Your challenges with food and body have not existed separately from any other part of you. "We are not going to solve these problems with the same patterns of domination and separation that created them," writes Sebene Selassie.[6] When you look around at your community and the leadership within it, who embodies equitable community and the relational focus needed to build something that invites us forward?

Body Trust Provider Carin Christy shared with us: "The most meaningful thing for me has come from being a part of a community where the active dismantling of the oppressive systems is welcomed, encouraged, and lived by the folks guiding the work."

There is community out here. You will not be alone, though you may feel lonely at times. It is not a perfect community, but it is a community. It's not perfect because we need more people who can embody their social location and do the work necessary to develop liberatory praxis and create communities that prioritize equity. And find ways to be together. So we use the tools we have. Social media is a place where you can find images of people who look like you living their big delicious lives unapologetically. You can curate your social media accounts so the only images you encounter support your healing and the expansion of the edges of your comfort zone regarding inclusion. Pursue doing the anti-racism and abolition work that you need to do. Look for affinity groups where you can come together and build connections based on shared identities or characteristics (fat, queer, BIPOC, trans, crip, etc.). Join body liberation groups on other platforms and go there to talk about how to move forward, how to care for your body, how to eat in a more attuned way, how to recover, but not to talk about your desire for weight loss or your latest food plan. Talking openly about weight or food plans in public places (including social media) ignores the inevitable impact on others who are listening. This stuff is never benign. It always has an impact on your community. There are always people recovering from eating disorders in your spaces. There are always people suffering in silence about their body story and body size. Our communities need fat affirmation, not diet talk.

It's an incredible thing to build a community around an idea that has taken root in you. These ideas turn into process and change and spark a necessity to keep going because it feels so right and is in alignment with who you are becoming. Communities that are built around healing, justice, and liberation are places we need. Many of us are still learning who to be together, and how to create a brave space while we wrestle with the presence of dominant culture. If we do not understand how shame moves through us, we are unlikely to rise to the occasion when we have done something to hurt someone else or we receive feedback that we are impacting someone negatively. We are all going to get it wrong sometimes, which is why Ericka Hines, founder of Black Womxn Thriving, says, "Be humble and ready to fumble." We want communities that are rooted in dignity, belonging, and a commitment to humanity. Love helps too.

In our Body Trust community, we often share this metaphor of how a colony of penguins helps each other by huddling together to survive in harsh conditions. Janaya Future Khan, cofounder of Black Lives Matter Toronto,[7] explains:

> Every time a penguin takes a step, all the other penguins have to shuffle with it in order to survive, so that the penguins on the inside are warm and the penguins on the outside are cold and they're gradually moving, and that's what care looks like. That's what community looks like. That's what thriving looks like. My wildest dream would be organizing our society not based on hierarchies, but based on spirals, based on care and community, based on knowing each other and knowing what each of us needs to get through. I think it's time for those on the margins to really shine.

Equitable community is where healing is possible. We heal in relationships. And our communities, which have commitments to equity and process, can hold the possibility of our liberation and healing.

We know you are likely surrounded by people who haven't been ready to listen to you or support your healing process. You may be wondering how you begin to share these ideas, or this newly developed aspect of your being, with them. Learning about Body Trust is like learning to speak a new language, and sometimes when you are fairly new in your own process and understanding of it, it can be especially hard to talk about. So we want share some of our thoughts with you. First, some conversation strategies:

Protect it. When starting this work, your roots are shallow because you are learning, so it may be best to protect this new thing for a while, and share it only with people who can hold space. As your roots deepen, it will be easier to hold your ground even when folks push back. You can say something like . . .

> *I'm exploring a radically different way of thinking about food, bodies, weight, and health. It's kind of blowing my mind, and I'm not sure I have words to talk about it just yet.*

Ask permission. When we ask people if we can share something with them, they are more likely to open up and hear it.

Acknowledge how different this work is. Saying that people bump up against *a lot* when they first hear about Health at Every Size, Body Trust, fat acceptance, or anti-diet approaches to food and eating is an understatement. If we prepare them, it may just help it land.

> *I want to acknowledge right up front that this is radically different from what we've been socialized to believe about bodies, weight, health, and fitness.*

Describe this growing community. Conjure up the community of people shouldering you in this work. You are not the only one. We are in this together. This may help you avoid second-guessing yourself and instead draw from the collective.

> *I'm learning from a growing community of people, which includes health care providers, researchers, academics, and*

helping professionals who are concerned about the health ef-
fects of the so-called obesity epidemic, and how the traditional
ways we've been taught to think about food, weight, and health
disrupt people's embodiment and negatively impact people's
ability to compassionately and sustainably care for themselves,
their bodies, and their communities.

Talk about how dieting has impacted your life negatively.
Share parts of your body story if and when you feel ready. People
are not allowed to argue with your lived experience.

Set boundaries. It's okay to ask for what you need. People may not
be able to hear it, and you can set a boundary.

You can do whatever you want with your life and your body,
and please honor and respect what I want to do with mine. I'd
like to ask that we not discuss bodies, food, health, or weight
when we are with each other. There are plenty of other things
we can talk about.

Share with people who are "reachable, teachable,
and ready." We learned this from Desiree Adaway and Ericka
Hines. There are just some folks who are never gonna get it
and will not be willing to even listen without debating and
exhausting you. Focus on folks who are reachable, teachable,
and ready.

"NO" and "STOP" are complete sentences. Sometimes there's
nothing more to say.

You may also be wondering what information to share that would
have the greatest impact. Here are a few of our go-to talking points:

* The body mass index has racist origins and was never intended to be used as a measure of health. It was developed by a mathematician in the nineteenth century to look at the distribution of weight across a population of white people. It is being used to stigmatize and pathologize people's bodies. BMI is not a vital sign.

* There's no evidence-based treatment for high body weight that leads to sustained weight loss two to five years out. The most consistent effect of weight loss at two years is weight gain.[8]

* There is research to show how weight stigma, racism, and other body-based oppressions, as well as other social determinants of health, have a far greater impact on our health and well-being than personal lifestyle behaviors. The truth is, lifestyle factors (health behaviors) actually account for 5 to 25 percent of the differences in health outcomes.[9] If we really care about people's health, we need to be fighting for things like racial justice, access to non-stigmatizing health care, living wages, clean air, affordable housing, and more.

* Emphasize how this work is about healing your relationship with food and body, not perfecting health behaviors. Body Trust helps people develop sustainable self-care behaviors instead of all the yo-yo dieting, yo-yo fitness, and weight cycling that diet culture enables, and research shows, negatively impact health. People are not required to pursue health to be deemed worthy of love, respect, and belonging.

The truth and the healing are in your story. Your story, unearthed, held, told despite shame, is the truth. It is evidence. And "We must leave evidence," writes Mia Mingus. "Evidence that we were here, that we existed, that we survived and loved and ached. Evidence of the wholeness we never felt and the immense sense of fullness we gave to each other. Evidence of who we were, who we thought we were, who we never should have been. Evidence for each other that there are other ways to live—past survival; past isolation."[10]

Early on, we asked you: What has come between you and being at home in your body? We wonder what your answer might be now, as we come to the end of this book. We hope, as this question reverberates through you, that you know your suffering has not been your fault. That Body Trust is your path. That you belong here. And that your body, in whatever size that it is, is you. Human, imperfect, changing, different than you wanted or ever expected, but nevertheless you. We ask you to remember, as you move forward, that fitting in will never be the same as belonging. You belong because you breathe. And that is enough.

We all have to step into the skin of the fiercely body compassionate to be free. So envision your freedom; assume it is for you and everyone else. Allow the softness to come. This will be a bold conversation in the current paradigm, but for those of us who hunger for truth and can intuit the path to freedom, it will be an ecstatic unveiling.

Additional Reading and Resources

There's as much to unlearn as there is to learn on the path to healing and liberation, and we see this book as one stepping-stone along the way. There are many amazing thought leaders, liberatory thinkers, teachers, and scholars in the world that we want you to know about, so we've created a webpage with recommended reading and resources to help you strengthen your analysis and deepen your roots into Body Trust. We have a directory of health care providers and helping professionals—our beloved Body Trust Provider community—who've trained with us and offer a variety of services to support you and your unique needs. You will also find a collection of journaling prompts to support each chapter in this book, a list of people and organizations to follow on social media, more body stories to read, and letters we've written to parents and caregivers, health care providers, and teachers and school administrators that we hope will be useful in your own life and advocacy work.

centerforbodytrust.com/reading-resources

Acknowledgments

We've been working together for seventeen years to build the language and philosophy that is Body Trust. We were business partners first, and as we and our work have grown and evolved, so has the depth of our friendship. We feel incredibly lucky to have found one another on this path and cannot imagine doing what we do without the other by our side.

We would first like to acknowledge that we have created this work on the traditional village sites of the Multnomah, Wasco, Cowlitz, Kathlamet, Clackamas, Bands of Chinook, Tualatin, Kalapuya, Molalla, and many other tribes who made their homes along the Columbia River in what has now come to be known as Portland, Oregon.

Our learning has primarily come through the people who have sat with us in our individual offices, groups, and workshops, and have shared their body stories with us. We remember you. And we thank you for bravely exploring something different instead of trying harder.

We are held and humbled by the solidarity and commitment of the people who have learned with us and call themselves Body Trust Providers. They both steward and expand the possibilities of this work beyond what we can imagine. Learn with them, hire them, trust them. Their commitment to liberatory approaches for bodies, to deep relationships, and to honoring lived experience may be exactly what you have been looking for.

We have shown up to and cultivated deep relationships with teachers who have allowed us to be seen and called in, trusted and held—who understand the interplay of love and power and meet us in both. Pamela Slim, Desiree Adaway, Ericka Hines, Jessica Fish, and Nicole Lee are the real deal in right relationship and we are grateful for their commitment to process. Ken Nelson was foundational in inspiring our curiosity about what it means to gather. We also acknowledge the teachers whom we do not know personally that are aiding in shaping and holding a vision of a liberatory future that keeps us in the day to day work: adrienne maree brown, Prentis Hemphill, Priya Parker, and many more.

We are grateful for the community of people we learned from and with early on: Lucy, Deb, Carol, Jane, Karin, Judith, Elyse, Evelyn, Sonya, Gloria, Marcella, and Amy. We offer a special acknowledgment to Barbara Meyer for being our initial collaborator in the Body Trust Network. The origin of the phrase Body Trust—as we understand it—is from dietitian Dayle Hayes in a video she produced called *Body Trust: Undieting Your Way to Health and Happiness* in 1993.

Body liberation work in helping or clinical spaces (such as Body Trust or Health at Every Size) is a professionalization of radical, grassroots, lifesaving activism by BIPOC and fat women and femmes who share in the origin story of the Fat Acceptance movement. These thought leaders, scholars, and teachers are the originators of this liberatory work and we are grateful for the sacrifices they made to share their wisdom and light with the world.

We are forever grateful for everyone who went before us, named the paternalistic and dominant threads woven through the healing professions, said "This is bullshit," and made something different. We also have endless gratitude for the committed generosity of Janell Mensinger, who has worked tirelessly to build a body of empirical evidence to support our Body Trust approach and bring this work to health care and eating disorder treatment.

This book was just a twinkle in our eye until we met Liz Bevilacqua at Storey Publishing. Liz helped us nurture a book proposal and then told us to take it into the world of publishing. Thank you, Pamela, for introducing us to our kind and fierce literary agent, Joelle Delbourgo, who helped us define this book project and ultimately connected us with Sara Carder and the team at TarcherPerigee who firmly believed in this book. We are grateful for the way you each helped us see the potential we were only holding a fraction of. Thank you, Sand Chang, for your contribution to this book, and Angela Braxton-Johnson, for the use of your poems. Thank you to the Body Trust participants who responded to our questionnaire, offered to be interviewed, and/or shared parts of your body stories with us for potential use in this book. And thank you, Jessica Davis, for reading our manuscript and offering us valuable insight and feedback that helped us improve this book and be ready to share it with the world.

And then there are the people who have their hands in Body Trust work every day, helping us make it all happen: Amanda Larson, we'd be lost without you! Dan Casey helps us communicate this paradigm to the world. We are forever grateful for your leadership and humanity. We are also thankful for Anna Chapman, Mary Stewart, and Amaya Villazan's contributions to our organization, and Kristi Moniatte for all your graphic design over the years. Your work is woven into the foundation of what we do. To the team at Wayward Kind and to Sirius Bonner for helping us envision the next phase of our business: The Center for Body Trust.

We appreciate those who have supported our well-being while writing this book and helped us keep going *and* growing: Carmen Cool, Chevese Turner, Lisa DuBreuil, Dawn Serra, Amy Frasieur. You are all walking the talk and we appreciate you.

Hilary would like to express love and gratitude to my family—Victor, Kyan, Luca, and my mom, Suzanne, for putting up with my constant doing and my weird and consuming work. Thank you for loving me enough to want this for me despite how it may have impacted you. I love you all. And to Carmen, Amanda, Desiree, and Amy for always being right there. I feel so human and enough in my relationships with you because of how you show up. I want to thank the people who support my well-being, such as Beth and Edie, and remind me that inclusive, relational health care is life-altering. I also want to thank my clients and my consultees. Thank you for trusting me with you and for allowing me to witness your beautiful, remarkable lives.

Dana would like to express love and gratitude to my husband, Oliver, parents, Darrell and Vicki, whose constant unwavering support of my personal and professional growth made so much of this possible. To my sisters, Mandalee and Weedster, for lifting me up, and my beloved French bulldog, Bosco, who was by my side most writing days. I miss your snuggles, snorts, snoring, and farts. Thank you, Beverly Glenn-Copeland, for writing songs that helped me trust my writing process and keep showing up to the work. Thank you, Jennifer, Rachael, Taryn, and Angela, for cheering me on and reminding me that I can do this. Thank you, Gaby and Edie, for supporting my well-being during the writing of this book. And to my beloved clients, you are my greatest teachers and I'm honored and humbled to be trusted to hold your story and your healing process.

Notes

Introduction

1. J. W. Anderson, E. C. Konz, R. C. Frederich, and C. L. Wood, "Long-term weight-loss maintenance: a meta-analysis of US studies." *The American Journal of Clinical Nutrition* 74, no. 5 (2001): 579–84. doi: 10.1093/ajcn/74.5.579.

2. T. Mann, A. J. Tomiyama, E. Westling, A. Lew, B. Samuels, and J. Chatman, "Medicare's search for effective obesity treatments: diets are not the answer." *American Psychologist* 62, no. 3 (2007): 220–33. doi: 1037/0003-066X.62.3.220.

3. W. C. Miller, "How effective are traditional dietary and exercise interventions for weight loss?" *Medicine & Science in Sports & Exercise* 31, no. 8 (1999): 1129–34. doi: 10.1097/00005768-199908000-0008.

4. Lucy Aphramor, "Effecting Change in Public Health," *Network Health Digest* 126 (2017): 55–59.

5. Dr. Linda Alvarez, "Colonization, Food, and the Practice of Eating," Food Is Power, https://foodispower.org/our-food-choices/colonization-food-and-the-practice-of-eating/.

6. Kerry Lusignan, "John Gottman and Brené Brown on Running Headlong into Heartbreak," The Gottman Institute, https://www.gottman.com/blog/john-gottman-and-brene-brown-on-running-headlong-into-heartbreak/.

7. Randi Buckley, "001: The Thing about You and Other People's Needs," June 19, 2019, produced by Randi Buckley, podcast, https://www.randibuckley.com/podcast-episodes/you-and-other-peoples-needs-001.

The Foundations of Body Trust

1. Prentis Hemphill, quoted with permission.

2. Tara Mohr, "The Good News About Your Inner Critic," https://www.taramohr.com/overcoming-self-doubt/the-good-news-about-your-inner-critic/.

3. Kristin D. Neff, Ya-Ping Hsieh, and Kullaya Dejitterat, "Self-compassion, achievement goals, and coping with academic failure," *Self and Identity* 4 (2005): 263–87, https://self-compassion.org/wp-content/uploads/publications/SClearninggoals.pdf.

4. Tara Brach, Resources, "RAIN: Recognize, Allow, Investigate, Nurture," https://www.tarabrach.com/rain/.

5. From Bobbie Harro, "The Cycle of Socialization," in *Readings for Diversity and Social Justice*, 4th ed., Maurianne Adams et al., eds. (New York: Routledge, 2018).

6. Virgie Tovar, "Lose Hate Not Weight," filmed July 19, 2017, TEDxSoMa video, 14:41, https://www.youtube.com/watch?v=hZnsamRfxtY.

Chapter 1: Body Trust Is a Birthright

1. Bobbie Harro, "The Cycle of Socialization," in *Readings for Diversity and Social Justice*, 4th ed., Maurianne Adams et al., eds. (New York: Routledge, 2018).

2. Medium, "The Making of 'Unruly Bodies,'" blog entry by Erica Spens, April 3, 2018, https://blog.medium.com/the-making-of-unruly-bodies-808dccb109e3.

3. Suzanne Pharr, *Homophobia: A Weapon of Sexism* (Oakland, CA: Chardon Press, 1988), p. 17.

4. Business Wire, "The $72 Billion Weight Loss & Diet Control Market in the United States, 2019–2023—Why Meal Replacements are Still Booming, but Not OTC Diet Pills—ResearchAndMarkets.com," February 25, 2019, https://www.businesswire.com/news/home/20190225005455/en/72-Billion-Weight-Loss-Diet-Control-Market.

5. T. Mann, A. J. Tomiyama, E. Westling, A. Lew, B. Samuels, and J. Chatman, "Medicare's search for effective obesity treatments: diets are not the answer." *American Psychologist* 62, no. 3 (2007): 220–33. doi: 1037/0003-066X.62.3.220.

6. J. W. Anderson, E. C. Konz, R. C. Frederich, and C. L. Wood, "Long-term weight-loss maintenance: a meta-analysis of US studies." *The American Journal of Clinical Nutrition* 74, no. 5 (2001): 579–84. doi: 10.1093/ajcn/74.5.579.

7. W. C. Miller, "How effective are traditional dietary and exercise interventions for weight loss?" *Medicine & Science in Sports & Exercise* 31, no. 8 (1999): 1129–34. doi: 10.1097/00005768-199908000-0008.

8. Susan Saulny, "Heavier Americans Push Back on Health Debate," *New York Times*, November 7, 2009, https://www.nytimes.com/2009/11/08/health/policy/08fat.html.

Chapter 2: Your Body Story

1. Aubrey Gordon, *What We Don't Talk About When We Talk About Fat* (Boston: Beacon Press, 2020), p. 137.

2. Lidia Yuknavitch (@LidiaYuknavitch), "I am not the story you made of me . . . ," Twitter, April 23, 2019.

3. Joey Keogh, "How Chrissy Metz Really Fells About Her Weight-Loss Contract," The List, March 26, 2020, https://www.thelist.com/196901/how-chrissy-metz-really-feels-about-her-weight-loss-contract/.

Body Trust and Trans Experience

1. E. W. Diemer, J. D. Grant, M. A. Munn-Chernoff, D. A. Patterson, and A. E. Duncan. "Gender identity, sexual orientation, and eating-related pathology in a national sample of college students." *Journal of Adolescent Health* 57, no. 4 (2015): 144–49, doi: 10.1016/j.jadohealth.2015.03.003.

Chapter 3: Your Coping Is Rooted in Wisdom

1. Savala Nolan, *Don't Let It Get You Down: Essays on Race, Gender, and the Body* (New York: Simon & Schuster, 2021), p. 181.

2. Durryle Brooks, "From Self-Care to Self-Reverence Practices: On Black People, Our Fight for Justice & Freedom," Medium, June 25, 2020, https://medium.com/@durryle.brooks/from-self-care-to-self-reverence-practices-on-black-people-our-fight-for-justice-freedom-72c962024a1b.

Chapter 4: Divesting from Diet Culture

1. Vanessa Rochelle Lewis, "Embracing Ugly in a World That's Tried to Weaponize It Against Me," Racebaitr, October 24, 2019, https://racebaitr.com/2019/10/24/embracing-ugly-in-a-world-thats-tried-to-weaponize-it-against-me/.

2. Marialaura Bonaccio et al., "High adherence to the Mediterranean diet is associated with cardiovascular protection in higher but not in lower socioeconomic groups: prospective findings from the Moli-sani study." *International Journal of Epidemiology* 46, no. 5 (2017): 1478–87, doi: 10.1093/ije/dyx145.

3. Your Fat Friend (Aubrey Gordon), "The Bizarre and Racist History of the BMI," Medium/Elemental Plus, October 15, 2019, https://elemental.medium.com/the-bizarre-and-racist-history-of-the-bmi-7d8dc2aa33bb.

4. Lindo Bacon and Lucy Aphramor, *Body Respect: What Conventional Books Get Wrong, Leave Out, and Just Plain Fail to Understand About Weight* (Dallas: BenBella Books, 2014), pp. 14–15.

5. Tracy L. Tylka et al., "The weight-inclusive versus weight-normative approach to health: evaluating the evidence for prioritizing well-being over weight loss." *Journal of Obesity* 2014, article ID 983495, doi: 10.1155/2014/983495.

6. T. Mann, A. J. Tomiyama, E. Westling, A. Lew, B. Samuels, and J. Chatman, "Medicare's search for effective obesity treatments: diets are not the answer." *American Psychologist* 62, no. 3 (2007): 220–33. doi: 1037/0003-066X.62.3.220.

7. Da'Shaun Harrison, *Belly of the Beast: The Politics of Anti-Fatness as Anti-Blackness* (Berkeley, CA: North Atlantic Books, 2021).

8. An Open, Digital Classroom on Gender, Intersectionality & Black Women's Rhetorics, "Social Construction of Gender," n.d., http://www.blackwomenrhetproject.com/why-must-we-remember-that-gender-is-socially-constructed-and-is-neither-a-binary-nor-a-biological-determination.html.

9. Reclaim UGLY, "Mission & Values," https://reclaimugly.org/about-us/.

10. Sand C. Chang, Anneliese A. Singh, lore m. dickey, *A Clinician's Guide to Gender-Affirming Care: Working with Transgender and Gender Nonconforming Clients* (Oakland, CA: Context Press, 2018), p. 10.

11. Sabrina Strings, *Fearing the Black Body: The Racial Origins of Fat Phobia* (New York: NYU Press, 2019), p. 6.

12. Naomi Wolf, *The Beauty Myth: How Images of Beauty are Used Against Women* (New York: Harper Perennial 2002), pp. 257–58.

13. E. W. Diemer, J. D. Grant, M. A. Munn-Chernoff, D. A. Patterson, and A. E. Duncan. "Gender identity, sexual orientation, and eating-related pathology in a national sample of college students." *Journal of Adolescent Health* 57, no. 4 (2015): 144–49, doi: 10.1016/j.jadohealth.2015.03.003.

14. Christy Harrison, "Food Psych #150: Disordered Eating & Gender Identity with Sand Chang," April 2, 2018, podcast, 1:25:23, https://christyharrison.com/foodpsych/5/eating-disorder-recovery-gender-identity-with-sand-chang#:~:text=Psychologist%20and%20trans%2Dhealth%20educator,nature%20of%20fatphobia%20and%20diet.

15. Read Sand Chang's letter "Dear Trans and Nonbinary Folks" on page 61 of this book.

16. Nick Bilton, "Hack the System: Tony Hsieh's Tragic Death Reveals the Dark Side of Silicon Valley's Biohacking Obsession," April 2021, https://archive.vanityfair.com/article/2021/4/hack-the-system.

17. Tracy L. Tylka et al., "The weight-inclusive versus weight-normative approach to health: evaluating the evidence for prioritizing well-being over weight loss." *Journal of Obesity* 2014, article ID 983495, doi: 10.1155/2014/983495.

18. Amanda Scriver, "This Photographer's Otherworldly Images Break Down How We Look at Different Bodies," *Brit + Co*, April 26, 2018, https://www.brit.co/this-photographers-otherworldly-images-break-down-how-we-look-at-different-bodies/.

Chapter 5: Reckoning with Your Eating

1. M. F. K. Fisher, *The Gastronomical Me* (New York: Duell, Sloan and Pearce, 1943).

2. Michael Twitty, "Michael Twitty on Culinary Justice | Observer Ideas," Guardian Live, October 30, 2014, YouTube video, 15:04. https://www.youtube.com/watch?v=EhxjC3XX54g.

3. Steven Bratman, MD, "Health Food Junkie," *Beyond Vegetarianism* (originally published in *Yoga Journal*, October 1997), https://www.beyondveg.com/bratman-s/hfj/hf-junkie-1a.shtml.

4. Tracy L. Tylka et al., "The weight-inclusive versus weight-normative approach to health: evaluating the evidence for prioritizing well-being over weight loss." *Journal of Obesity* 2014, article ID 983495, doi: 10.1155/2014/983495.

5. Ellyn Satter, *Secrets of Feeding a Healthy Family: How to Eat, How to Raise Good Eaters, How to Cook*, 2nd ed. (Madison, WI: Kelcy Press, 2008), p. 1.

6. Lindsey Bever, "A Hungry Gwyneth Paltrow Fails the Food-Stamp Challenge Four Days In," *Washington Post*, April 17, 2015, https://www.washingtonpost.com/news/morning-mix/wp/2015/04/17/a-hungry-gwyneth-paltrow-fails-the-food-stamp-challenge-four-days-in/.

7. Jennifer Crowley, Lauren Ball, and Gerrit Jan Hiddink, "Nutrition in medical education: a systematic review." *The Lancet* 3, no. 9 (2019): e379–e389, doi: 10.1016/S2542-5196(19)30171-8.

8. Carolyn Becker, Keesha Middlemass, Francesca Gomez, and Andrea Martinez-Abrego, "Eating disorder pathology among individuals living with food insecurity: a replication study." *Clinical Psychological Science* 7, no. 5 (2019), doi: 10.1177/2167702619851811.

9. Ellyn Satter Institute, How to Eat, "The Joy of Eating: Being a Competent Eater," 2022, https://www.ellynsatterinstitute.org/how-to-eat/the-joy-of-eating-being-a-competent-eater/.

10. Isabel Abbott, from a September 19, 2018 Facebook post, used with permission.

11. Jane Hirshmann and Carol Munter were the first to write about this concept in their book, *Overcoming Overeating: Conquer Your Obsession with Food* (New York: Ballantine Books, 1966).

12. FoodShare, Body Positivity Statement, https://foodshare.net/about/body-positivity/.

Chapter 6: What Does Grief Have to Do with It?

1. Lama Rod Owens, "An Informal Contemplation on Healing," Mountain Record, Summer/Fall 2018, https://www.mountainrecord.org/bfod/remembering-love/#.

2. Savala Nolan, *Don't Let It Get You Down: Essays on Race, Gender, and the Body* (New York: Simon & Schuster, 2021), p. 180.

3. Elisabeth Kübler-Ross, *On Death and Dying* (London: Tavistock Publications, 1969).

4. "Let's Talk About Grief," Amazing Care Network, December 18, 2018, https://www.amazingcarenetwork.com/lets-talk-about-grief/.

5. Meredith Noble, "Body Acceptance Begins with Grieving the Thin Ideal," Made on a Generous Plan, https://www.generousplan.com/body-acceptance-grieving-thin-ideal/.

6. David Whyte, "Anger," in *Consolations: The Solace, Nourishment and Underlying Meaning of Everyday Words* (Langley, WA: Many Rivers Press, 2014).

7. Tanya Geisler, "In the Spotlight with Tanya Geisler, Featuring Staci Jordan Shelton," May 18, 2017, 26:16, https://tanyageisler.com/blog/itsstaci.

8. Jeanne Courtney, "Size acceptance as a grief process: observations from psychotherapy with lesbian feminists." *Journal of Lesbian Studies* 12, no. 4 (2008): 347–63, doi: 10.1080/10894160802278218, https://pubmed.ncbi.nlm.nih.gov/19042744/.

9. Angela Braxton-Johnson, "I Woke Up Like That," November 2017; originally published in *Unchaste Anthology*, vol. 2, Jenny Forrester, ed. (Portland, Ore.: Unchaste Press, 2017). For more information, see angelabraxtonjohnson.com.

Chapter 7: Ending the Hustle

1. Pete Walker, "Shrinking the Inner Critic," http://pete-walker.com/shrinkingInnerCritic.htm.

2. "United States' Weight Loss Market to Decline by 9% to $71 Billion in 2020—Assessment of the Changing Consumer Dieting Behavior Due to COVID-19," PR Newswire, June 4, 2020, https://www.prnewswire.com/news-releases/united-states-weight-loss-market-to-decline-by-9-to-71-billion-in-2020—-assessment-of-the-changing-consumer-dieting-behavior-due-to-covid-19-301070748.html.

3. Stasha Smiljanic, "19+ Statistics and Facts about the Fitness Industry (2021)," Policy Advice, February 14, 2021, https://policyadvice.net/insurance/insights/fitness-industry-statistics/.

4. "Global Cosmetic Skin Care Industry (2020 to 2027)—Market Trajectory & Analytics," GlobeNewswire, September 25, 2020, https://www.globenewswire.com/news-release/2020/09/25/2099275/0/en/Global-Cosmetic-Skin-Care-Industry-2020-to-2027-Market-Trajectory-Analytics.html.

5. Leah Lakshmi Piepzna-Samarasinha, "A Not-So-Brief Personal History of the Healing Justice Movement, 2010–2016," *MICE Magazine*, n.d., https://micemagazine.ca/issue-two/not-so-brief-personal-history-healing-justice-movement-2010%E2%80%932016.

6. Jennifer Brady, Jacqui Gingras, and Lucy Aphramor, "Theorizing health at every size as a relational-cultural endeavour." *Critical Public Health* 23, no. 3 (2013) 345–55, doi: 10.1080/09581596.2013.797565.

7. Caleb Luna (@chairbreaker) "On Fat Embodiment & Divesting from Constructions of Health," Instagram post from July, 10, 2020, https://www.instagram.com/p/CCeoUfdAFZw/.

8. Leah Lakshmi Piepzna-Samarasinha, *Care Work: Dreaming Disability Justice* (Vancouver, BC: Arsenal Pulp Press, 2018), p. 123.

9. Aubrey Gordon, *What We Don't Talk About When We Talk About Fat* (Boston: Beacon Press, 2020), p. 158.

Meg's Body Story

1. Mary Oliver, "The Summer Day," from *New and Selected Poems* (Boston: Beacon Press, 1992).

Chapter 8: Entering the Wilderness

1. Elizabeth Gilbert, *Big Magic: Creative Living Beyond Fear* (New York: Riverhead Books, 2015), p. 247.

2. Brené Brown, "The Gifts of Imperfection," Courage, https://brenebrown.com/art/tgoi-sacred-ground/.

3. Niva Piran, *Journeys of Embodiment at the Intersection of Body and Culture: The Developmental Theory of Embodiment* (Cambridge, MA: Academic Press, 2017), p. 11.

4. Rosemary Faire, Somatic Intelligence (2002), Somatic Literacy, http://somaticliteracy.com/.

5. Shoog McDaniel, About, http://shoogmcdaniel.com/about.

6. makespacecounselling, from a March 25, 2021, Instagram post quoting @shooglet, https://www.instagram.com/p/CM1pAoiLZKv/.

7. heydrsand, from a June 28, 2021, Instagram post, https://www.instagram.com/p/CQrXDG2LWQm/.

8. "She Majestic Tree," Angela Braxton-Johnson, © July 2018. For more information, see angelabraxtonjohnson.com.

Chapter 9: Allowing for Pleasure and Satisfaction

1. adrienne maree brown, *Pleasure Activism: The Politics of Feeling Good* (Chico, CA: AK Press, 2019), p. 433.

2. Brené Brown, "Shame resilience theory: a grounded theory study on women and shame." *Families in Society: The Journal of Contemporary Social Services* 87, no. 1 (2006): 43–52. doi: 10.1606/1044-3894.3483.

3. Carmen Cool, @carmencool, "The goal of therapy should never be to help people adjust to oppression." tumblr, July 26, 2018, https://fleshengineer.tumblr.com/image/178512994996.

4. Angel Dunbar, "Black Pain, Black Joy, and Racist Fear: Supporting Black Children in a Hostile World," Psychology Benefits Society, August 30, 2017, https://psychologybenefits.org/2017/08/30/encouraging-black-childrens-self-expression/.

5. Brené Brown, "The Power of Vulnerability," filmed June 2010, in Houston, TX, TEDx video, 20:03, https://www.ted.com/talks/brene_brown_the_power_of_vulnerability.

6. Mark Matousek, "Unlocking Erotic Intelligence: Advice from Esther Perel," *Psychology Today*, March 29, 2013, https://www.psychologytoday.com/us/blog/ethical-wisdom/201303/unlocking-erotic-intelligence-advice-esther-perel.

7. Audre Lorde, "The Uses of the Erotic: The Erotic as Power," chapter 5 in *Sister Outsider: Essays and Speeches*, Audre Lorde, ed. (Berkeley, CA: Crossing Press, 1984), p. 88.

Chapter 10: Reclaiming Movement

1. Finding Our Hunger Podcast "UNradical" with Virgie Tovar, Episode 143, March 28, 2016, https://www.stitcher.com/show/finding-our-hunger/episode/unpodcast-143-unradical-virgie-tovar-finding-our-hunger-43422047.

2.   Ilya Parker, "What Is Toxic Fitness Culture?" Decolonizing Fitness, June 17, 2020, https://decolonizingfitness.com/blogs/decolonizing-fitness/what-is-toxic-fitness-culture.

3.   Christine Byrne, "How to Tell if Your Relationship with Exercise Is Actually Toxic," *Huff Post*, August 23, 2021, https://www.huffpost.com/entry/how-to-tell-if-relationship-exercise-toxic_l_5efb3f86c5b612083c52ff7d.

4.   Fringeish, Instagram post on May 17, 2021, https://www.instagram.com/p/CO-fM-utCIQ/.

5.   V. W. Barry, M. Baruth, M. W. Beets, J. L. Durstine, J. Liu, S. N. Blair, "Fitness vs. fatness on all-cause mortality: a meta-analysis." *Progress in Cardiovascular Diseases* 56, no. 4 (2014): 382–90, doi: 10.1016/j.pcad.2013.09.002.

6.   Aubrey Gordon and Michael Hobbes, "The President's Physical Fitness Test," The Maintenance Phase, October 20, 2020, 58:00, https://podcasts.apple.com/us/podcast/the-presidents-physical-fitness-test/id1535408667?i=1000495386842.

7.   Niva Piran, *Journeys of Embodiment at the Intersection of Body and Culture: The Developmental Theory of Embodiment* (Cambridge, MA: Academic Press, 2017), pp. 7–8.

8.   Piran, *Journeys of Embodiment at the Intersection of Body and Culture.*

9.   National Eating Disorders Association, "Compulsive Exercise," https://www.nationaleatingdisorders.org/learn/general-information/compulsive-exercise.

Chapter 11: Deepening Your Roots into Body Trust

1.   Sonya Renee Taylor, *The Body is Not an Apology: The Power of Radical Self-Love* (Oakland, CA: Berrett-Koehler Publishers, 2018), p. 79.

2.   Danna Faulds, from "Sangha," in *Go In and In: Poems from the Heart of Yoga* (Berkeley, CA: Peaceable Kingdom Press, 2002).

3.   Kerry Lusignan, "John Gottman and Brené Brown on Running Headlong into Heartbreak," The Gottman Institute, https://www.gottman.com/blog/john-gottman-and-brene-brown-on-running-headlong-into-heartbreak/.

4.   samdylanfinch, Instagram post from June 9, 2020, https://www.instagram.com/p/CBO3llNjg5G/.

5.   Evelyn Tribole and Elyse Resch, *Intuitive Eating: A Revolutionary Anti-Diet Approach*, 4th ed. (New York: Macmillan, 2020), p. 150.

6.   We adapted these steps from the helpful book by Cristien Storm, *Living in Liberation: Boundary Setting, Self-Care and Social Change* (Port Townsend, WA: Feral Book Press, 2010), pp. 43–49.

7.   Jane R. Hirschmann and Carol H. Munter, *When Women Stop Hating Their Bodies: Freeing Yourself from Food and Weight Obsession* (New York: Ballantine Books, 1996).

Chapter 12: Making Your Healing Bigger Than You

1. Mary Oliver, "The Summer Day."

2. Judy Freespirit and Aldebaran, "Fat Liberation Manifesto," *Off Our Backs* 9, no. 4 (April 1979): 18, https://www.jstor.org/stable/25773035?refreqid=excelsior%3A77 3802e746f7f97ae11bea9af54188d2.

3. bell hooks, *All About Love: New Visions* (New York: William Morrow, 1999), p. 215.

4. Niva Piran, *Journeys of Embodiment at the Intersection of Body and Culture: The Developmental Theory of Embodiment* (Cambridge, MA: Academic Press, 2017), pp. 6–7.

5. Piran, *Journeys of Embodiment at the Intersection of Body and Culture*, pp. 25–26.

6. "Feeling Disconnected? Here's How to Connect and Belong with Sebene Salassie," Real Food Whole Life, https://realfoodwholelife.com/feelgoodeffect/connect-belong-sebene-selassie/.

7. stylelikeu, Instagram post from August, 5, 2021, https://www.instagram.com/p/CSNIVQXhfpP.

8. Tracy L. Tylka et al., "The weight-inclusive versus weight-normative approach to health: evaluating the evidence for prioritizing well-being over weight loss." *Journal of Obesity* 2014, article ID 983495, doi: 10.1155/2014/983495.

9. Lucy Aphramore, PhD, "Effecting Change in Public Health," *Network Health Digest* 126 (2017): 55–59.

10. Leaving Evidence, About, https://leavingevidence.wordpress.com/about-2/.

Index

Note: Italicized page numbers indicate material in tables or illustrations.

About the Authors

Hilary Kinavey is a politicized therapist, coach, and educator whose work has focused on shifting the way we interact with and care for bodies—our own and others. She supports health care professionals in doing system-challenging radical care work. She lives with her partner and two children, her therapy dog in training, beautiful cats, and a lot of wild waterfowl, just outside of Portland, Oregon.

Dana Sturtevant is a radical dietitian and educator whose work is focused on humanizing health care, advancing health equity, and advocating for food and body sovereignty. She is passionate about music, loves to dance like nobody's watching, and is happiest when close to the ocean or a waterfall. She lives in Portland, Oregon, with her husband and rescue dog.

The Center for Body Trust offers e-courses, workshops, and retreats for people to explore Body Trust in community, as well as training programs for helping professionals and educators interested in adopting client-centered, trauma-informed, justice-based approaches to healing—including an intensive year-long training to become a Body Trust Provider. Their work has been featured in the *New York Times*, *Scientific American*, *Health*, *Self*, *Real Simple*, *Huffington Post*, and on the TEDx stage. Learn more at centerforbodytrust.com.